A Rheumatologist's Guide to
INTERPRETING IMAGING
IN SPONDYLOARTHRITIS

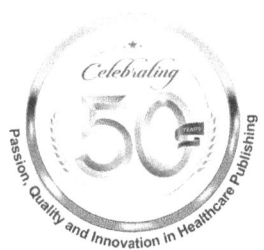

A Rheumatologist's Guide to INTERPRETING IMAGING IN SPONDYLOARTHRITIS

Authors

Ashish Sharma
MBBS MD (Internal Medicine) Fellowship Rheumatology
Consultant
Department of Rheumatology
Fortis Hospital
Noida, Uttar Pradesh, India

Vivek Arya
MBBS MD (Internal Medicine)
Consultant
Department of General Medicine and Rheumatology
North Devon District Hospital
Barnstaple, UK

Abhinetri KSV
MBBS MD (Radiodiagnosis)
Consultant
Department of Radiology
Fortis Flt Lt Rajan Dhall Hospital
New Delhi, India

Foreword
Ashok Kumar

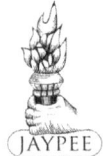

JAYPEE BROTHERS MEDICAL PUBLISHERS
The Health Sciences Publisher
New Delhi | London

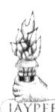 **Jaypee Brothers Medical Publishers (P) Ltd**

Headquarters

Jaypee Brothers Medical Publishers (P) Ltd
4838/24, Ansari Road, Daryaganj
New Delhi 110 002, India
Phone: +91-11-43574357
Fax: +91-11-43574314
E-mail: jaypee@jaypeebrothers.com

Overseas Office

JP Medical Ltd
83 Victoria Street, London
SW1H 0HW (UK)
Phone: +44 20 3170 8910
Fax: +44 (0)20 3008 6180
E-mail: info@jpmedpub.com

Website: www.jaypeebrothers.com
Website: www.jaypeedigital.com

© 2020, Jaypee Brothers Medical Publishers

The views and opinions expressed in this book are solely those of the original contributor(s)/author(s) and do not necessarily represent those of editor(s) of the book.

All rights reserved. No part of this publication may be reproduced, stored or transmitted in any form or by any means, electronic, mechanical, photocopying, recording or otherwise, without the prior permission in writing of the publishers.

All brand names and product names used in this book are trade names, service marks, trademarks or registered trademarks of their respective owners. The publisher is not associated with any product or vendor mentioned in this book.

Medical knowledge and practice change constantly. This book is designed to provide accurate, authoritative information about the subject matter in question. However, readers are advised to check the most current information available on procedures included and check information from the manufacturer of each product to be administered, to verify the recommended dose, formula, method and duration of administration, adverse effects and contraindications. It is the responsibility of the practitioner to take all appropriate safety precautions. Neither the publisher nor the author(s)/editor(s) assume any liability for any injury and/or damage to persons or property arising from or related to use of material in this book.

This book is sold on the understanding that the publisher is not engaged in providing professional medical services. If such advice or services are required, the services of a competent medical professional should be sought.

Every effort has been made where necessary to contact holders of copyright to obtain permission to reproduce copyright material. If any have been inadvertently overlooked, the publisher will be pleased to make the necessary arrangements at the first opportunity. The **CD/DVD-ROM** (if any) provided in the sealed envelope with this book is complimentary and free of cost. **Not meant for sale.**

Inquiries for bulk sales may be solicited at: jaypee@jaypeebrothers.com

A Rheumatologist's Guide to Interpreting Imaging in Spondyloarthritis

First Edition: **2020**

ISBN: 978-93-89776-95-9

Contributors

Ashok Kumar
MBBS MD (Internal Medicine) FRCP (London)
Director and Head
Department of Rheumatology
Fortis Flt Lt Rajan Dhall Hospital
Vasant Kunj, New Delhi, India
Formerly, Professor and Head of Rheumatology
Department of Medicine
AIIMS, New Delhi, India

Bimlesh Dhar Pandey
MBBS MD (Internal Medicine) MRCP
Consultant
Department of Rheumatology
Fortis Hospital
Noida, Uttar Pradesh, India

Mohammad Ali
MBBS MD (Internal Medicine)
Medical Officer
Department of Medicine
Atal Bihari Vajpayee Institute of Medical Sciences
and Dr Ram Manohar Lohia Hospital
New Delhi, India

Foreword

Diagnostics of spondyloarthritis have come a long way. The driving force behind this development is obviously the availability of highly effective anti-TNF drugs. The classical 'bamboo-spine' is encountered uncommonly in present day practice owing to diagnosis of spondyloarthritis at a much earlier stage. Imaging plays a crucial role in early diagnosis.

Dr Ashish Sharma is a bright young rheumatologist with keen interest in medical imaging. At the same time, he is an excellent rheumatologist. Dr Vivek Arya is an eminent Professor of General Medicine and consultant rheumatologist in the UK. Dr Abhinetri is an astute radiologist with special interest in musculoskeletal imaging. The three authors have produced this book in which they have illustrated a variety of radiographs, MRIs and CT scans of patients with spondyloarthritis. Many of the imaging features, which we seldom see (or notice!), have been nicely presented in the form of high quality pictures.

Spondyloarthritis is far beyond sacroiliac joints, is a fact this book brings out very well, including changes in the ligaments, which can easily be seen on plain radiographs. Although MRI is very sensitive in identifying acute changes in spondyloarthritis, it also picks up nonspecific changes, which need proper interpretation. The authors provide a balanced approach, which utilizes plain radiography and MRI optimally. I frequently come across anxious patients coming to me for a second opinion, with an MRI report (which looks quite scary!). It is very unusual to find an absolutely 'normal' MRI report. Overindulgence in MRI frequently leads to erroneous diagnoses. That is why it is very important for rheumatologists to have a basic understanding of MRI, so that they can interpret the films themselves, keeping in view all the clinical parameters.

The authors have explained the science of MRI in very simple manner and have thoroughly explained various findings on MRI in patients with spondyloarthritis. This will definitely help clinicians in broadening their horizon to look beyond sacroiliac joints and to interpret the findings themselves, rather than relying on the MRI report! This book will help our radiology colleagues too in better understanding non-traumatic, musculoskeletal imaging, where the experience in radiology is relatively suboptimal.

CT scan is just an extension of plain radiographs and has limited utility in spondyloarthritis. Chronic structural changes are better visualized on CT. Fractures of the spine occur frequently in patients with spondyloarthritis because of the high prevalence of spinal osteoporosis in them. Such occult fractures are a frequent cause of disabling pain in AS patients and are better picked-up on CT. Not uncommonly, clinicians interpret spinal pain as evidence of active AS and miss the occult fracture of spine.

I am sure this book will be an excellent guide for clinicians in interpreting imaging in patients with spondyloarthritis. The book demonstrates how to get the best out of both plain radiography and MRI in diagnosing spondyloarthritis. MRI has a definite role in non-radiographic spondyloarthritis. It should be interpreted in a mature way, taking into consideration the clinical features and acute phase reactants. The book has the potential to create a healthy change in the manner spondyloarthritis imaging is utilized and interpreted in clinical practice. In addition, it is also a valuable resource for both clinicians and rheumatologists.

Ashok Kumar MBBS MD FRCP (London)
Director and Head
Department of Rheumatology
Fortis Flt Lt Rajan Dhall Hospital
Vasant Kunj, New Delhi
Formerly, Professor and Head of Rheumatology
Department of Medicine, AIIMS
New Delhi, India

Preface

This book is meant for the practicing rheumatologist. It will also be useful for postgraduate students and internists with an interest in Rheumatology. It intends to familiarize clinicians involved in the care of patients with spondyloarthritis (SpA) with various common and uncommon imaging features of these disorders. In addition, it will serve as a reference for comparison of imaging features observed by clinicians in their day-to-day practice.

We have presented various imaging features of SpA on radiographs, MRI and CT scans. Besides hip, knee and ankle joints, other peripheral joints have not been included, like interphalangeal joints, which are commonly involved in psoriatic arthritis. Moreover, various mimics of SpA on imaging have not been included, as they are out of the scope of this book.

Imaging in SpA is not just about the sacroiliac joints. Many other features are to be looked into, as described in the book. Plain radiographs are an excellent modality for detecting structural changes. Moreover, structural progression can be easily monitored by radiographs due to their easy reproducibility in terms of cost and radiation exposure. MRI is very helpful in detecting active inflammation. Moreover, inflammation at various entheseal sites and the presence of chronic changes (fatty metaplasia, erosions, sclerosis, and ankylosis) can be very helpful in making a correct diagnosis of SpA in cases where classification criteria for SpA are not met but the clinical suspicion is high.

Clinico-radiological correlation is indispensable for making a correct diagnosis, which is best possible if the imaging plates are read by the treating physicians themselves.

Our aim is not to make rheumatologists into radiologists or to do away with the role of a radiologist in interpreting imaging related to SpA. Far from it, this is a collaborative work involving both rheumatologists and a consultant radiologist.

The purpose is to make it easier for a rheumatologist to understand the report given by a radiologist in this context and to participate with a basic understanding during multidisciplinary meetings involving radiology colleagues. The ultimate aim is to ensure better patient care through shared understanding of imaging findings.

We hope the reader will enjoy reading this book as much as we have enjoyed writing it!

Ashish Sharma
Vivek Arya
Abhinetri KSV

Contents

1. Introduction 1
2. Radiographs 6
3. MRI of Sacroiliac Joint 31
4. MRI of Spine 45
5. Infections Mimicking SpA 52
6. MRI of Peripheral Joints 55
7. Hip Joint Arthritis and Avascular Necrosis of Hip 65
8. CT Scan 68
9. Abbreviations 73
10. References 74

INTRODUCTION

Imaging plays an important role in the diagnosis, management and follow-up of patients with spondyloarthropathies and has been an integral component of the classification criteria for spondyloarthritis (SpA). Modified New York criteria (1984),[1] Amor criteria (1990/1991)[2] and the European Spondyloarthropathy Study Group criteria (ESSG) (1991)[3] used radiographs for defining sacroiliitis. A major limitation of radiographs is the inability to detect early inflammatory lesions, before the structural damage has occurred. Magnetic resonance imaging (MRI) has emerged as an excellent imaging modality which, in addition to the chronic structural changes, can also detect active/ongoing inflammatory changes early in the disease course. This has led to earlier diagnosis of SpA in patients with inflammatory back pain (IBP) and timely initiation of treatment, thereby preventing structural damage. In 2009, The Assessment of Spondyloarthritis International Society (ASAS) laid down the classification criteria for axial-SpA which included MRI in the imaging arm of the criteria, which had never been used in the earlier criteria.[4] With the use of MRI, non-radiographic axial-SpA has emerged as an important entity.[5]

Sacroiliitis is the most characteristic feature of axial-SpA. There are 4 grades of sacroiliitis on plain radiographs of pelvis, according to the severity (discussed further). Appearance of sacroiliitis on MRI depends on its stage – acute or chronic. Four types of acute lesions in sacroiliac joint (SIJ) have been described – bone marrow edema (also called osteitis), synovitis, capsulitis and enthesitis. Similarly, there exist four types of chronic lesions – fatty metaplasia, erosions, sclerosis and ankylosis.[6]

Sacroiliac joint has an upper ligamentous part and lower cartilaginous part (Fig. 1).[7] The ligamentous part connects ilium and sacrum with the help of strong ligaments and lacks synovial membrane. So it is not a true synovial joint and hence no inflammation of the joint occurs in this part. But, enthesitis can occur involving the ligaments present in this part of SIJ (*see* Fig. 47). The lower cartilaginous part is the true synovial joint with the presence of hyaline articular cartilage, synovial membrane and joint capsule. Thus, it is the lower cartilaginous part of the SIJ where true sacroiliitis occurs.

Conventional radiography is an inexpensive and well-established imaging technique. Anteroposterior projection of the X-ray of pelvis with the patient in supine position and the

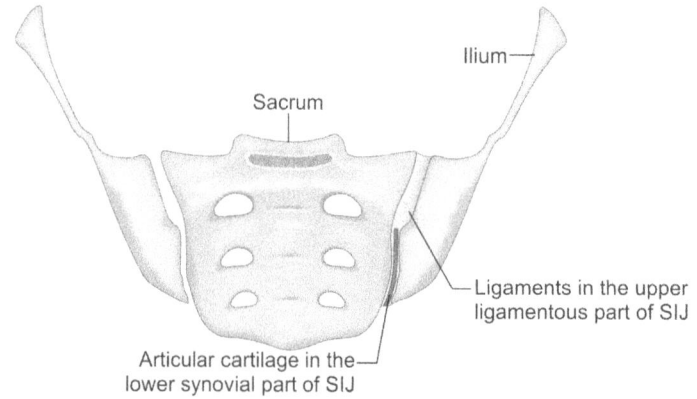

Fig. 1: Anatomy of the SIJ, showing the upper ligamentous part and lower synovial part. (SIJ: sacroiliac joint).

tube angulated 15–30° in the cephalad direction is considered appropriate for imaging the SIJ.[8] In addition, radiographs of the cervical, thoracic and lumbar spine should be obtained in anteroposterior and lateral projections. Although the Modified Stoke Ankylosing Spondylitis Spine Score (mSASSS)[9] includes only cervical and lumbar spine in the evaluation of structural changes, it is advisable to image the thoracic spine also because of the presence of prominent structural changes in this part of the spine (*see* Fig. 16).

Computed tomography (CT) helps in better visualization of the structural changes such as erosions and new bone formation, in axial, sagittal and coronal planes as compared to radiographs, but early inflammatory changes cannot be detected.

Among the various imaging modalities, MRI is the only modality that can depict both active inflammatory and structural changes, as well as their anatomical distribution. A field strength of at least 1.5 Tesla should be used in the evaluation of SpA.[10] Out of the various sequences of MRI, T1 weighted and short tau inversion recovery (STIR) sequences are sufficient for imaging the SIJ.[11] The images of the SIJ must be obtained in the oblique coronal plane, parallel to the long axis of the sacrum, and in the axial plane. T1 and T2 sequences are fat-sensitive, which means that fat appears bright on these sequences. Bone marrow is composed of fat in addition to the hematopoietic tissue and the proportion of fat in the marrow increases with age. T1 sequence, being fat-sensitive, provides a good contrast between the bright marrow fat and dark cortical line. Due to this, erosions are best visualized on T1.[6,10] On the other hand, STIR sequence inherently suppresses fat and gives bright signal with water.[10] Therefore, inflammation/marrow edema appears bright against a dark marrow signal due to the suppression of marrow fat. T2 weighted sequences do not have much role in the imaging of SpA unless the images are fat-suppressed (fat-suppressed T2W sequence give similar images as STIR) since both, the inflammation and fat, appear bright.

Sacroiliitis on radiographs is defined by the Modified New York criteria (Table 1).[1,12] Four grades of sacroiliitis have been described. Grade-1 is the mildest grade of sacroiliitis with doubtful changes on the radiograph and a high degree of inter-observer variability. Grade-2 is suggestive of definite sacroiliitis which is defined by the presence of sclerosis of articular margins of SIJ and the subarticular bone in the presence of normal joint space. As soon as the width of joint space gets altered, it is termed grade-3. Joint space can either be widened (due to extensive erosions) or narrowed (due to sclerosis of joint margins). Grade-4 sacroiliitis is the most severe form where there is obliteration of the joint space due to bony ankylosis. Ankylosis can either be patchy or may involve the whole of SIJ. Spine radiographs are helpful in visualizing the structural changes which include erosions at the corner of the vertebral bodies (also called Romanus lesions).[13,14] As the corner erosions heal, sclerosis occurs which

Table 1: Grades of radiographic sacroiliitis. For defining AS according to modified New York criteria, there should be either bilateral grade-2 sacroiliitis or unilateral grade-3 or 4 sacroiliitis.[1]

Grade	Joint space	Additional features
1	Normal	Doubtful changes
2	Normal	Definite changes - sclerosis of joint margins
3	Widened or narrowed	Sclerosis, erosions
4	Obliterated	

appear on radiographs as radiopaque shadows in the corners of the vertebral bodies (shiny-corner sign).[13] Squaring is the straightening of anterior border of the vertebral bodies due to calcification of the anterior longitudinal ligament. Calcification of annulus fibrosus of the intervertebral discs leads to the formation of syndesmophytes. Latter can be either bridging or non-bridging depending on whether the calcification of annulus is complete or not, respectively. In addition, sclerosis and erosions of the vertebral endplates, disc calcifications, bony bridging, intervertebral ankylosis and ossification of various spinal ligaments can be seen in SpA.

Magnetic resonance imaging is extremely capable of depicting the active bone marrow edema or osteitis earlier than conventional radiography or CT, thus aiding in the early detection of SpA. Bone marrow edema is the earliest stage of inflammation which appears in the subchondral zone of the cartilaginous part of the SIJ.[6] It is considered as an essential criterion for defining sacroiliitis on MRI according to the ASAS criteria. It appears on MRI as bright signal on STIR and dark signal on T1. Synovitis appears as a bright intense signal on STIR within the SIJ cavity. Synovitis cannot be visualized on T1 sequence, but on injection of contrast, the inflamed synovium shows contrast enhancement and gives a bright signal. Similarly, capsulitis appears bright on STIR and contrast-enhanced T1 sequences, best appreciated in the coronal section at the superior edge of the SIJ. Enthesitis may be seen as bright signal intensity of the tendinous insertions with associated bone marrow edema at the underlying site of attachment of the entheses. Use of contrast in SpA imaging is of no added advantage. It leads to enhancement of acute lesions, which can also be visualized on STIR without contrast injection.[15] Moreover, contrast injection increases the cost and time taken for the MRI and it cannot be used in patients with derangement of renal function.

After the resolution of bone marrow edema, the area involved gets replaced by fat as an attempt towards healing. This is called fatty metaplasia and appears bright on T1 and dark on STIR. Fatty infiltration begins from the subchondral part of the SIJ and progresses medially. This may lead to an appearance of a bright signal on STIR at the periphery of the fatty lesion, representing resolving bone marrow edema (*see* Fig. 39).[11] Erosions are best visualized on T1 sequence appearing as defects in the bony outline. Sclerosis gives dark signal on all the sequences and is not enhanced by contrast injection. Ankylosis gives rise to obliteration of the joint space of SIJ. It can be patchy, involving only a part of the SIJ or may be extensive involving the whole of the SIJ. All the lesions can also be seen at other sites including spine and peripheral joints.

In the spine, inflammation appears in the form of bone marrow edema at the corners of the vertebral bodies (called spondylitis).[13] Spondylitis appears bright on STIR and is seen at anterior and posterior corners of the vertebrae. Spondylitis can lead to erosions, which appear dark on T1, and these lesions are the MRI counterpart of radiographic Romanus lesions. Spondylitis may also heal with fatty metaplasia at the corners (also called fatty Romanus lesions). Ultimately sclerosis of the corners may occur, giving rise to dark signals on all the sequences, which is the MRI counterpart of radiographic shiny corner sign.

Different lesions may appear similar on different sequences of MRI. For example, a bright lesion in the subarticular region of SIJ is bone marrow edema on STIR images and fatty metaplasia on T1. Bone marrow edema suggests active disease which requires appropriate treatment. On the other hand, fatty metaplasia may not be associated with active disease, but is a lead indicator of radiographic progression. However, it may not require aggressive treatment. Thus, it is necessary to identify the sequence of MRI. Fat is the most important component that helps us in identifying the sequence of MRI. If the area of the subcutaneous fat is bright, then it is either T1 or T2. STIR suppresses fat strongly, so the subcutaneous area appears dark. In the MRI of the SIJ, it is helpful to look at the urinary bladder. If the content of the urinary bladder appears dark, then it is a T1W image. Urine appears bright on T2W images and STIR. Another way of differentiation is the visualization of the intervertebral discs and cerebrospinal fluid. Nucleus pulposus has high water content, which makes the central portion of the discs appear bright on T2W and STIR images and dark on T1W images. Similarly, the cerebrospinal fluid in the spinal canal appears dark on T1W images and bright on T2W and STIR images. In the presence of bright cerebrospinal fluid or urinary bladder, if the subcutaneous fat appears bright, then it is T2W image, otherwise it is either fat-suppressed T2 or STIR sequence.

In this book, we illustrate and discuss various features of SpA on different modalities of imaging. This book aims to serve as a guide to rheumatologists in interpretation of individual imaging features of SpA. The images have been collected during routine outpatient care of patients with SpA or suspected SpA, with their informed consent.

RADIOGRAPHS

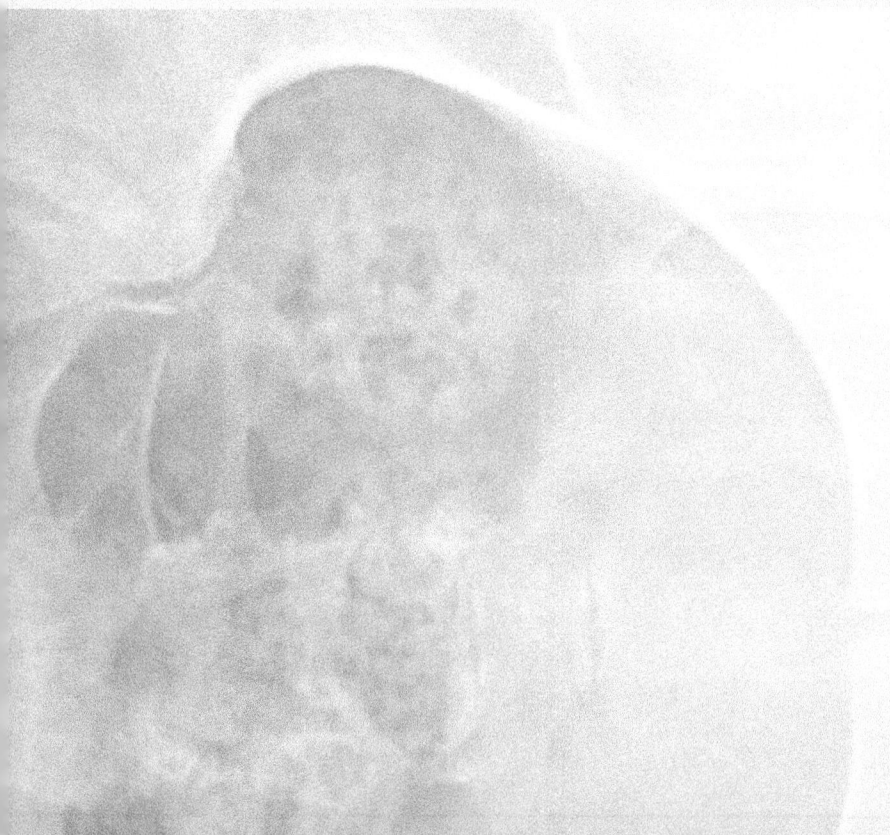

Radiographs

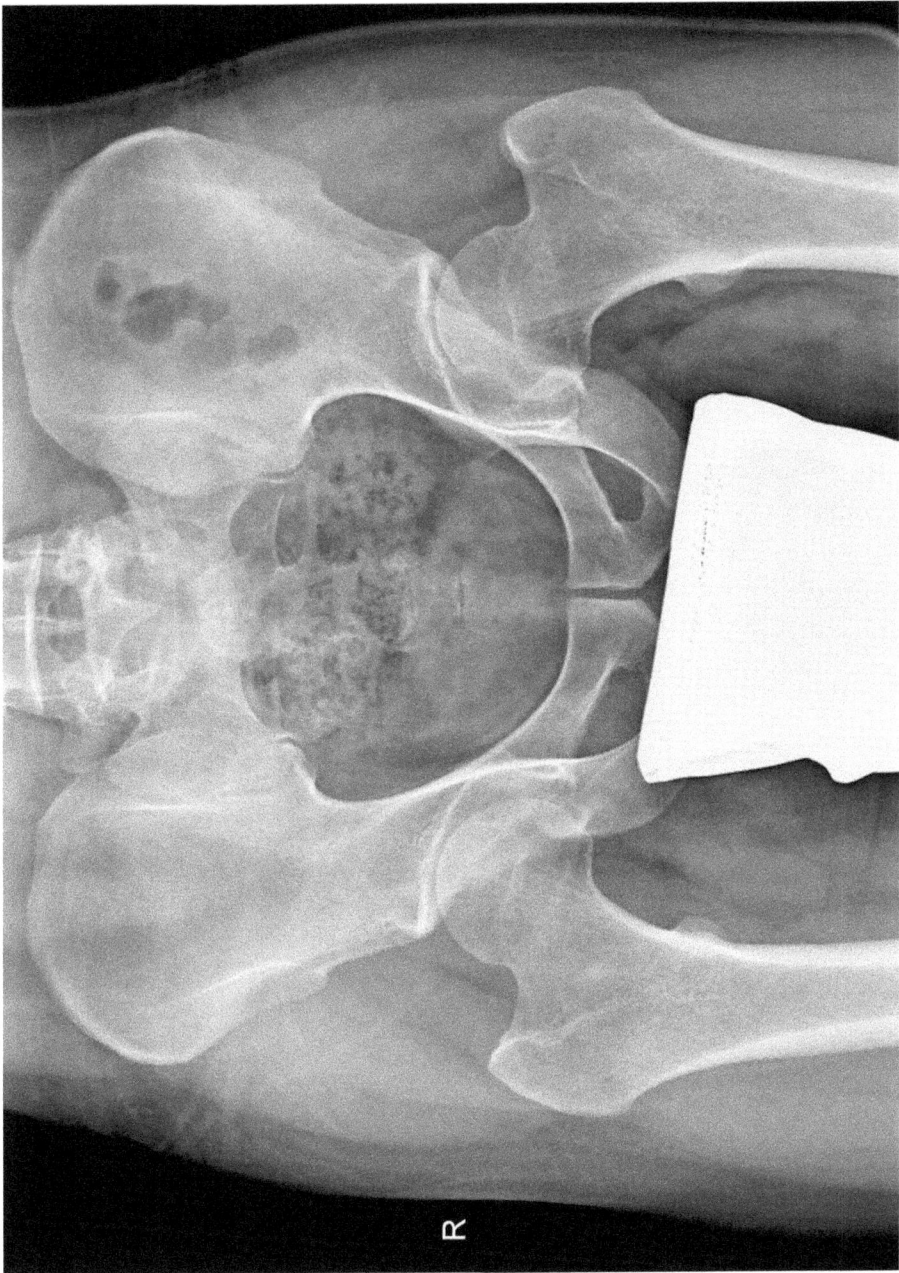

Fig. 2: Radiograph of pelvis, anteroposterior projection showing a normal SIJ with regular joint margins, normal joint space and no sclerosis around the joint line. Hip joints and all the entheseal sites are normal.

8 A Rheumatologist's Guide to Interpreting Imaging in Spondyloarthritis

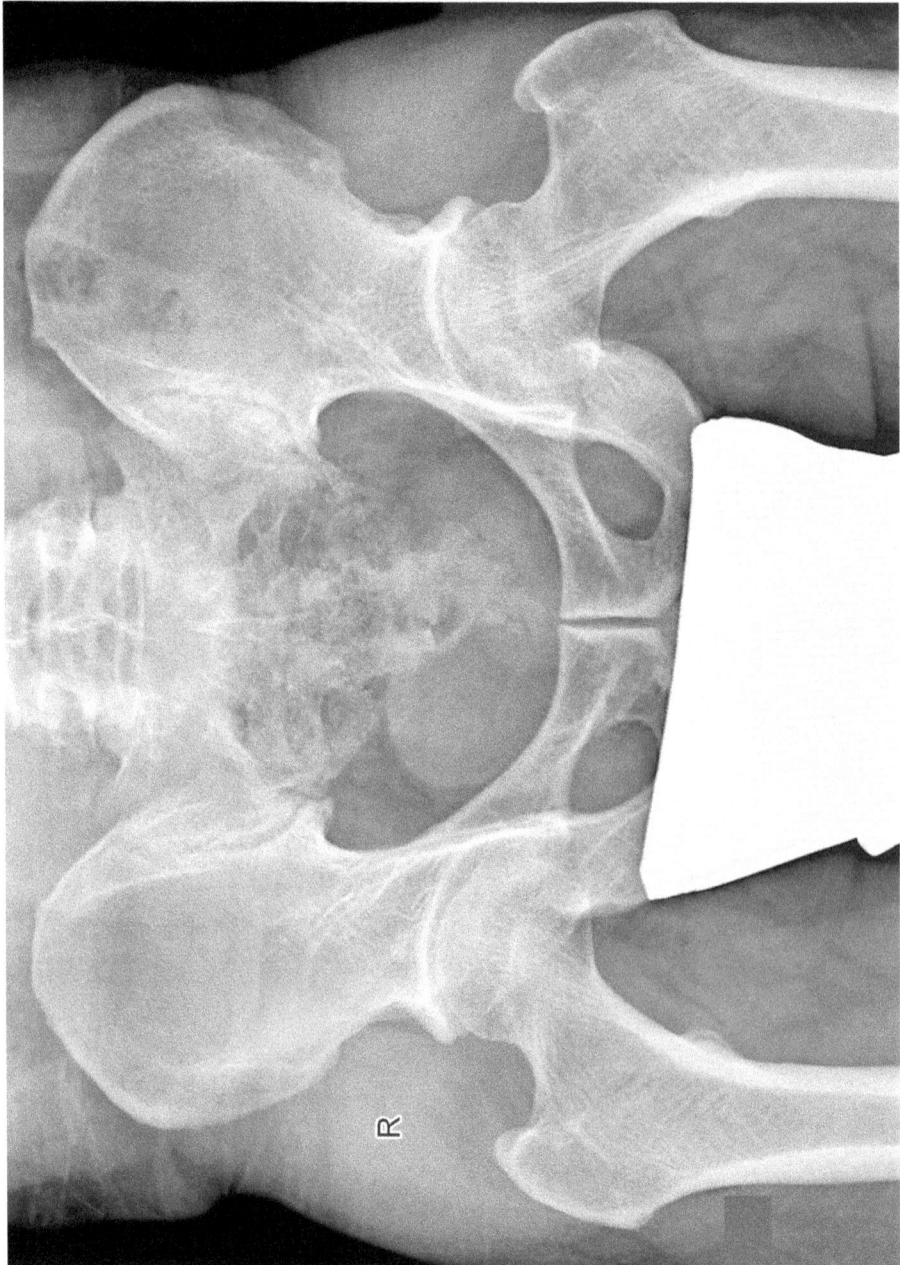

Fig. 3: Radiograph of pelvis, anteroposterior projection showing sclerosis of the joint margins of right SIJ with normal joint space (grade-2 sacroiliitis). In addition to periarticular sclerosis, there is irregularity of joint margins and narrowing of the joint space in left SIJ (grade-3 sacroiliitis).

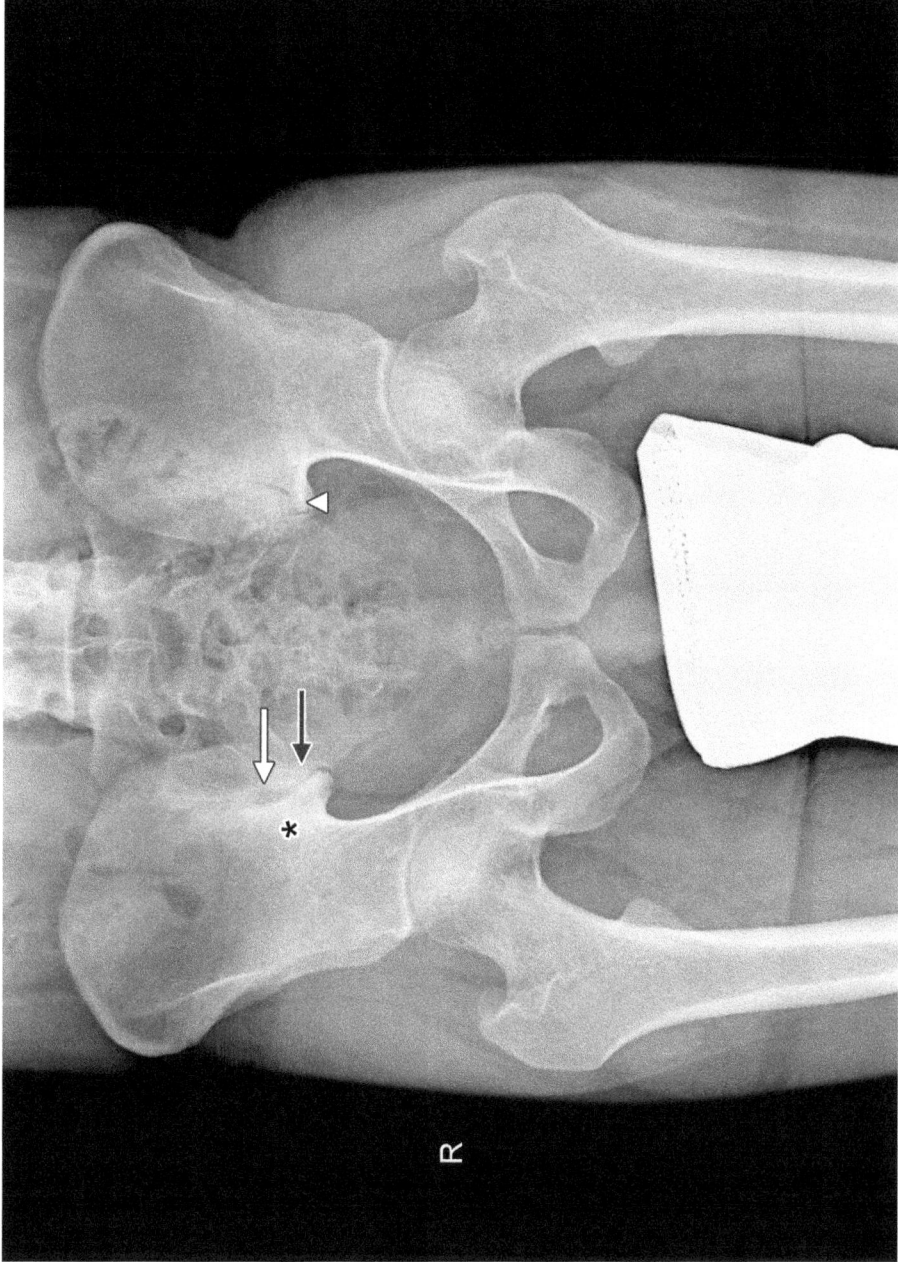

Fig. 4: Radiograph of pelvis, anteroposterior projection showing periarticular sclerosis of right SIJ (asterisk) with widening of the lower part of joint space (white arrow) with narrowing of joint space in the lowest part of right SIJ (black arrow) [grade-3 sacroiliitis]. Lowest part of left SIJ shows mild sclerosis (arrowhead) [grade-1 sacroiliitis].

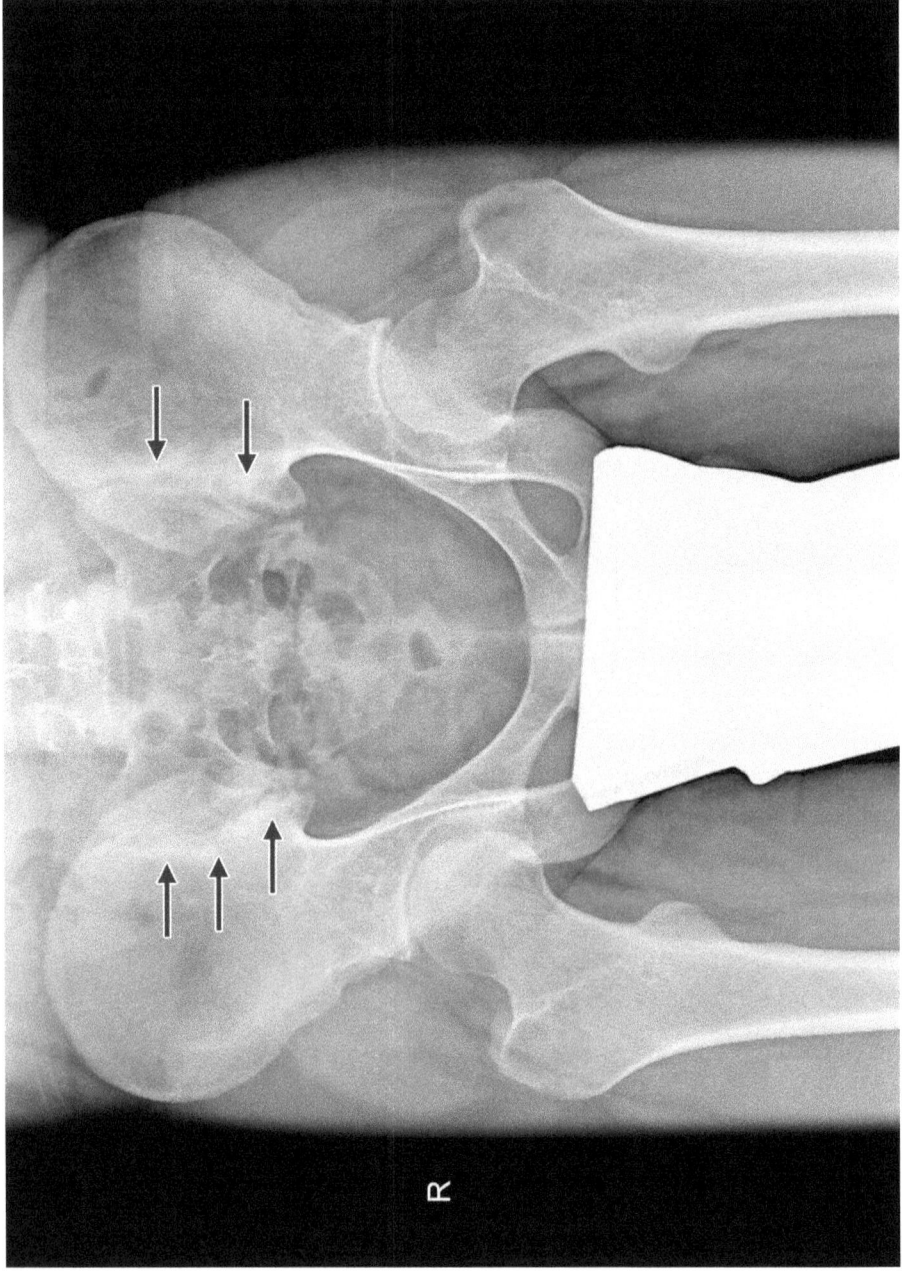

Fig. 5: Radiograph of pelvis, anteroposterior projection showing periarticular sclerosis (arrows) and irregular joint margins in both SIJ (grade-3 sacroiliitis).

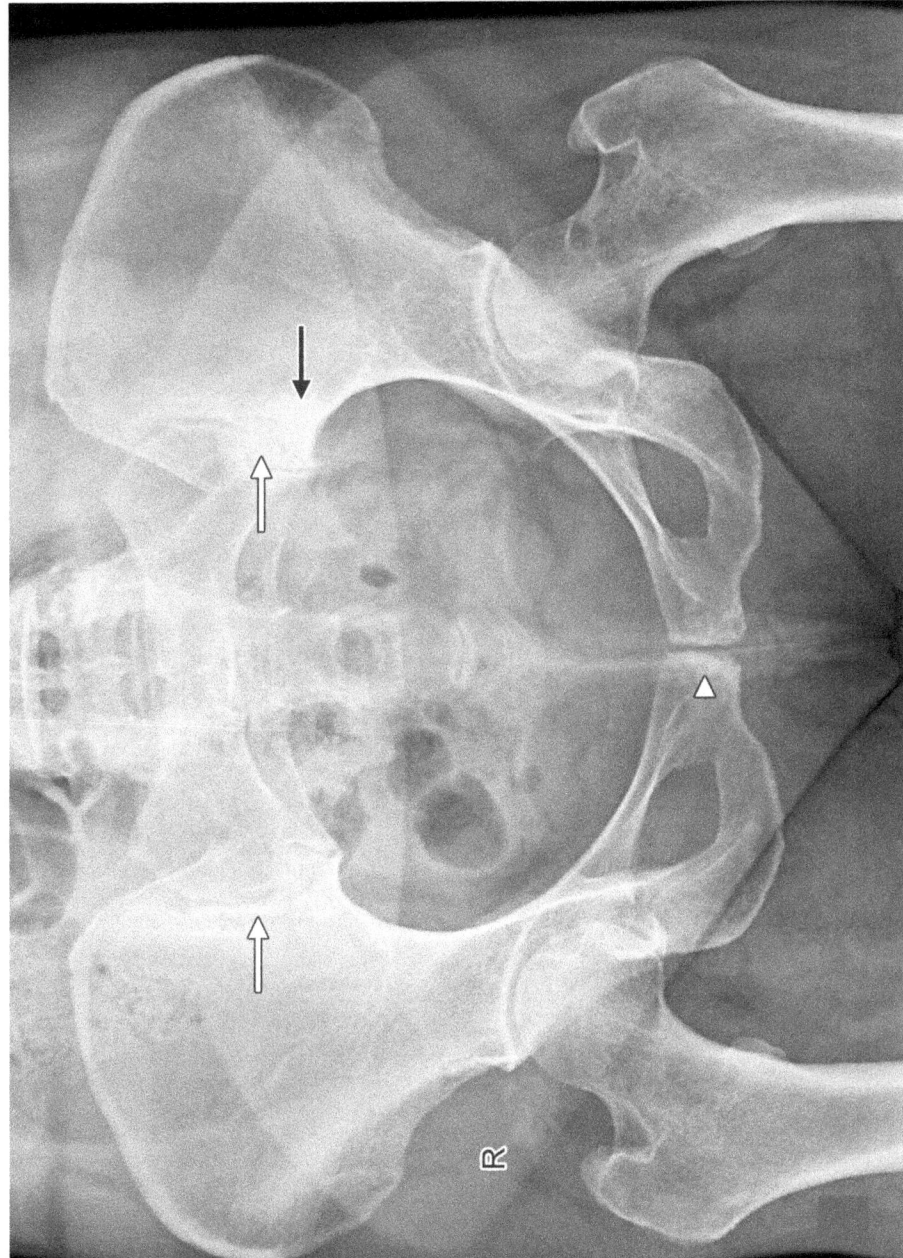

Fig. 6: Pelvic radiograph, anteroposterior projection of a multiparous 40-year old lady with AS showing periarticular sclerosis in right SIJ (white arrow) [grade-2 sacroiliitis]; sclerosis (white arrow) and narrowed joint space in left SIJ (grade-3 sacroiliitis). Note the triangular-shaped radiodensity in the ilium extending away from the left SIJ, suggestive of osteitis condensans ilii (black arrow). It is identified by its peculiar triangular shaped radiodensity and can be mistaken for inflammatory sacroiliitis. Sclerosis is also observed in pubic symphysis, more on right side (arrowhead).

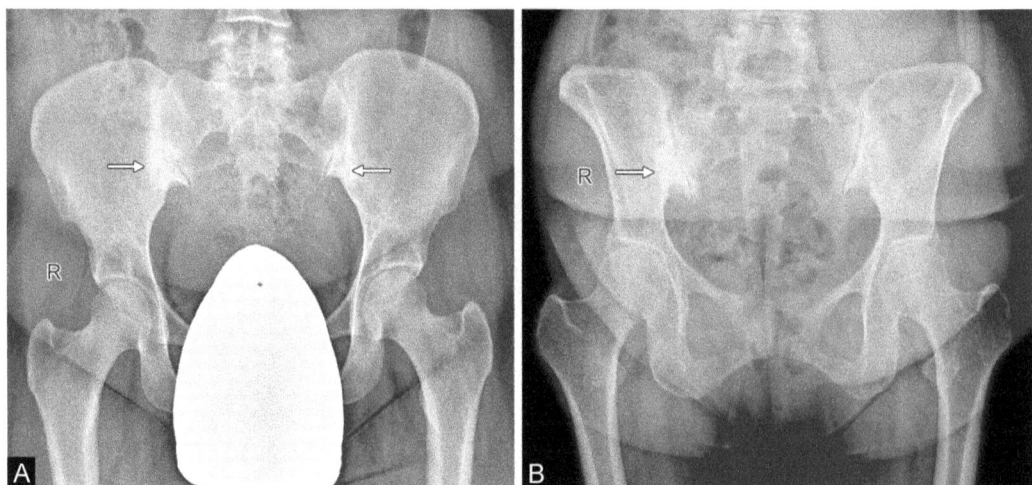

Figs. 7A and B: Radiographs of pelvis, anteroposterior projection showing radiodensity along the iliac aspect of SIJ extending away from the joint (white arrows), suggestive of osteitis condensans ilii (bilateral in A, right sided in B).

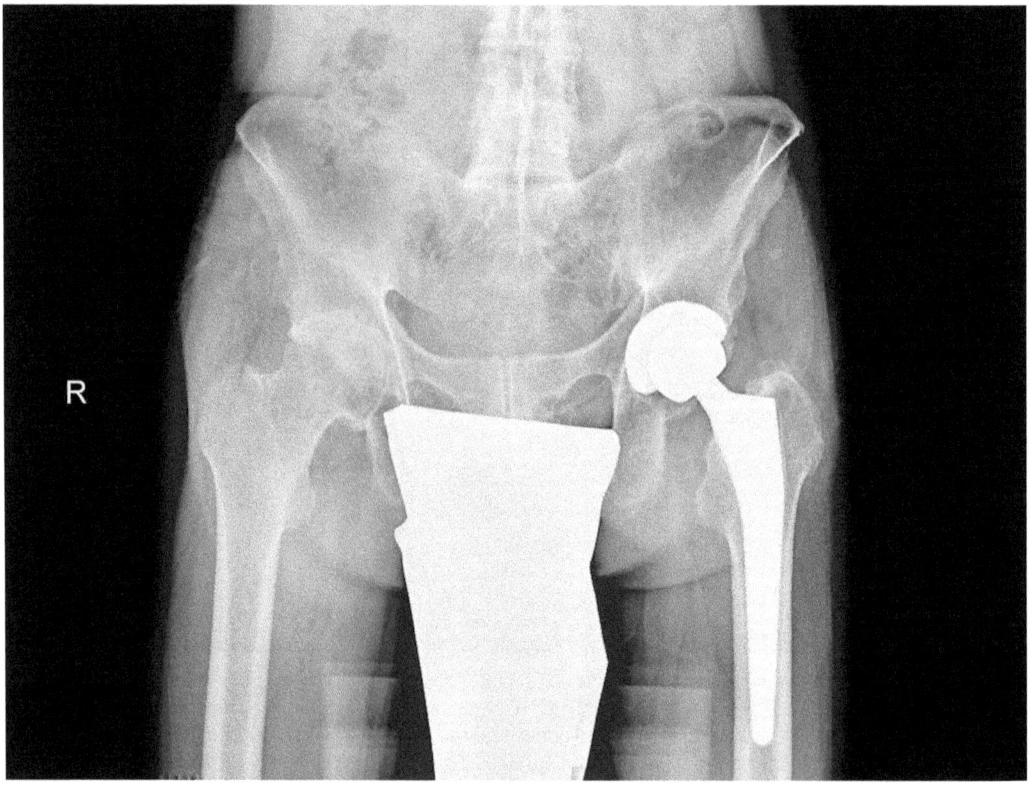

Fig. 8: Radiograph of pelvis, anteroposterior projection showing obliterated (ankylosed) SIJ on both sides (grade-4 sacroiliitis), reduced joint space of right hip, total hip replacement prosthesis on the left side due to severe damage of left hip joint (hip arthritis is a marker of severe disease in SpA).

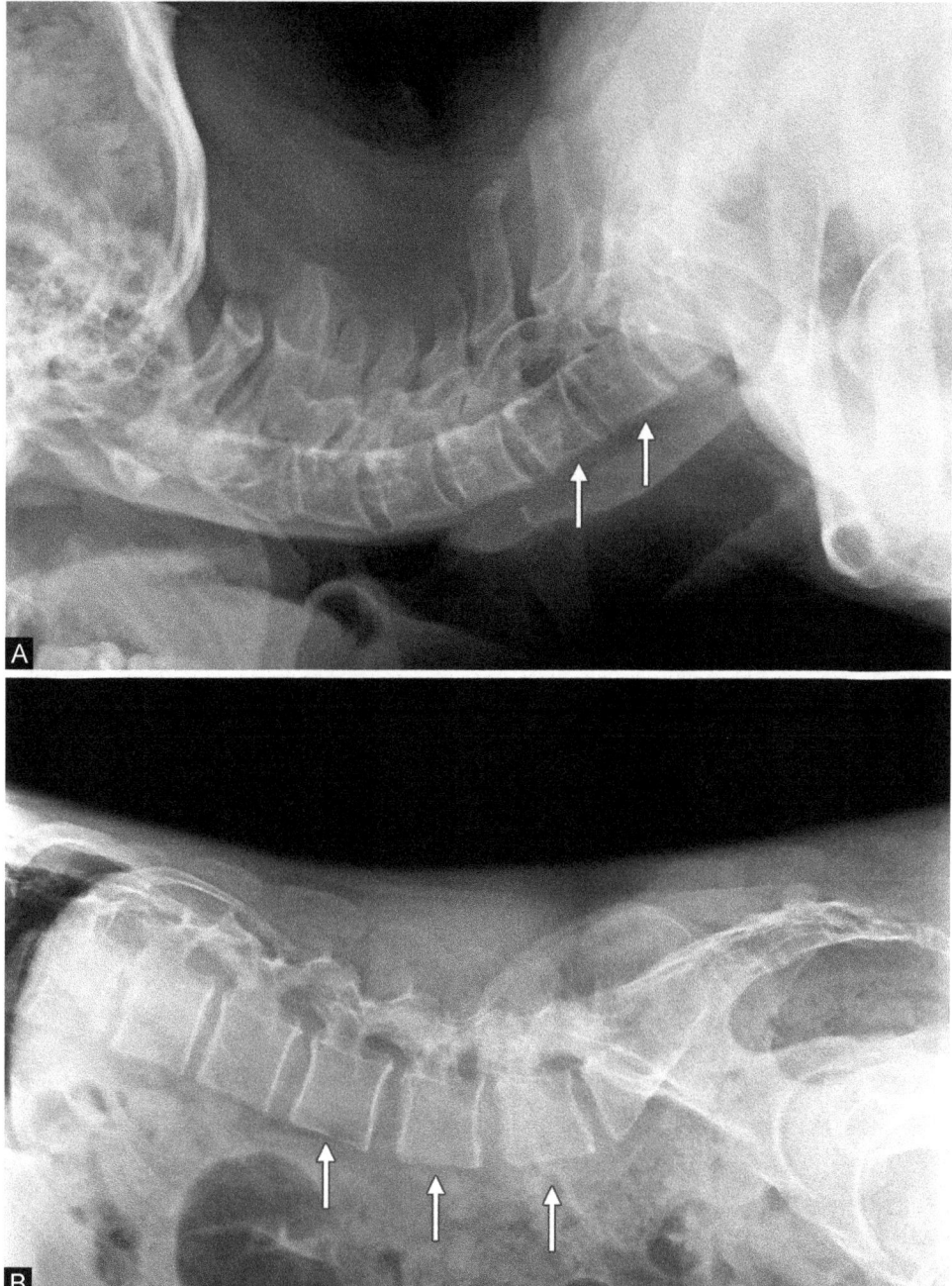

Figs. 9A and B: Radiographs of the cervical (A) and lumbar spine (B), lateral projections showing loss of normal concavity with straightening of the anterior borders of the vertebral bodies, suggestive of squaring (white arrows).

A Rheumatologist's Guide to Interpreting Imaging in Spondyloarthritis

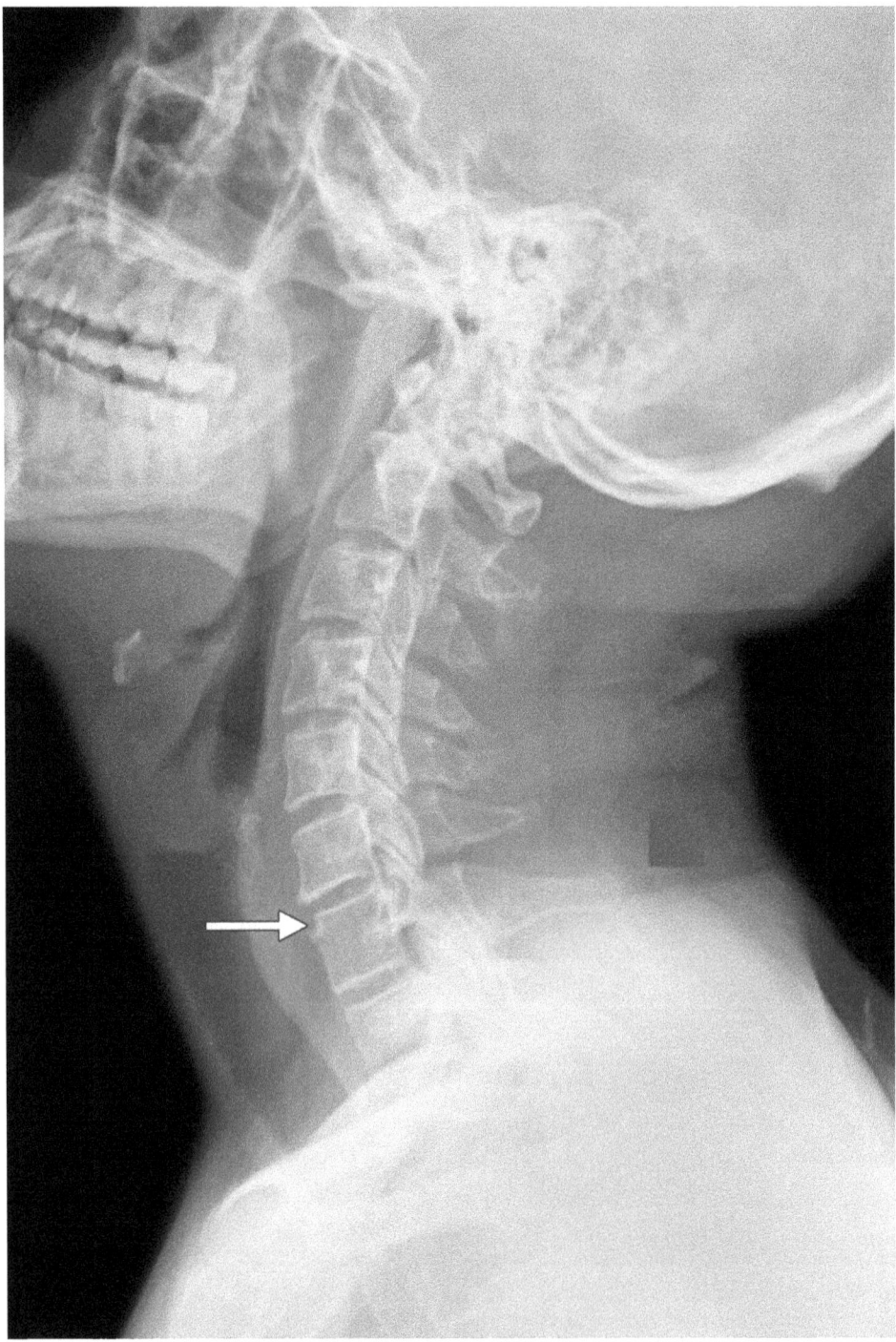

Fig. 10: Radiograph of cervical spine, lateral projection showing erosion of the anterior upper corner of C7 vertebra: Romanus lesion (arrow).

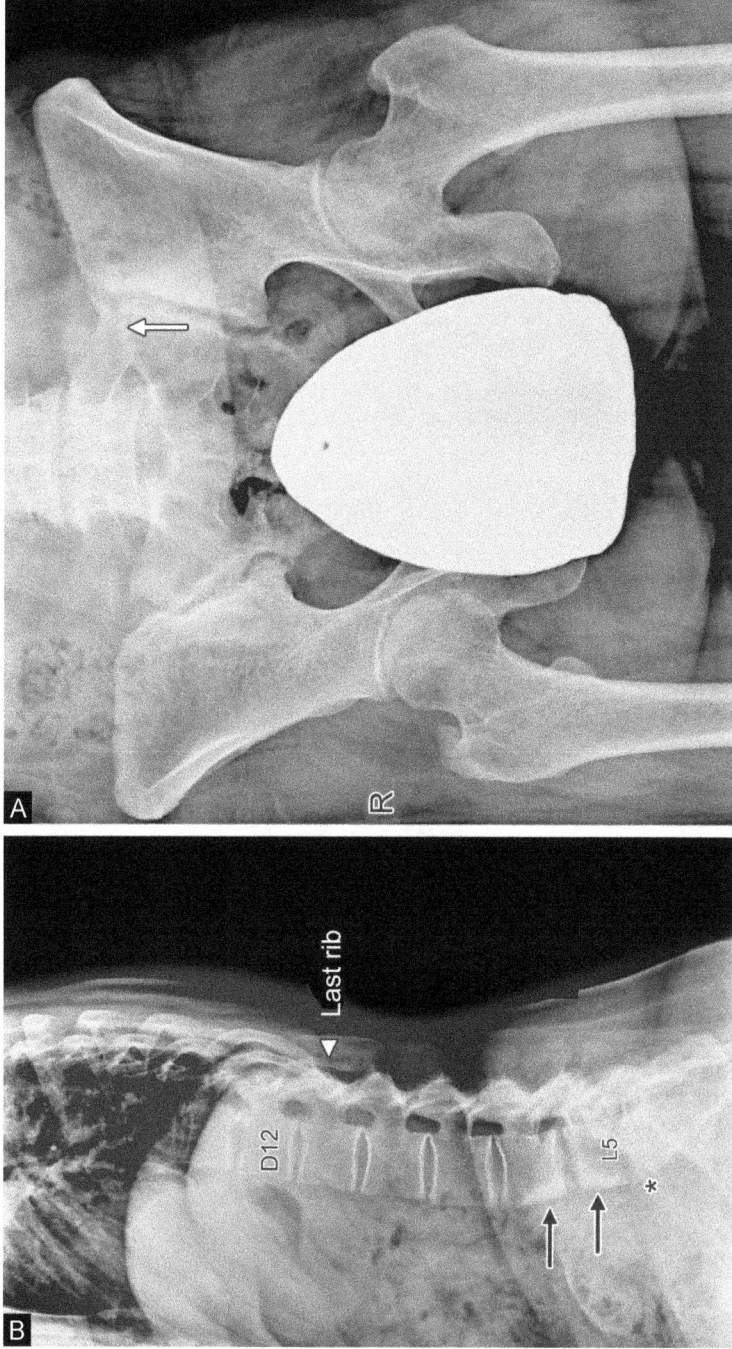

Figs. 11A and B: (A) Radiograph of pelvis, anteroposterior projection showing widening of both SIJ (grade-3 sacroiliitis) and pseudoarticulation of the left transverse process of L5 with the ala of sacrum (transitional vertebra) (white arrow); (B) Radiograph of thoracolumbar spine, lateral projection of the same patient showing sclerosis of lower anterior corner of L4 and upper anterior corner of L5 ('shiny' corner sign) (black arrows). Note partial sacralization of L5 (asterisk), leading to formation of transitional vertebra.

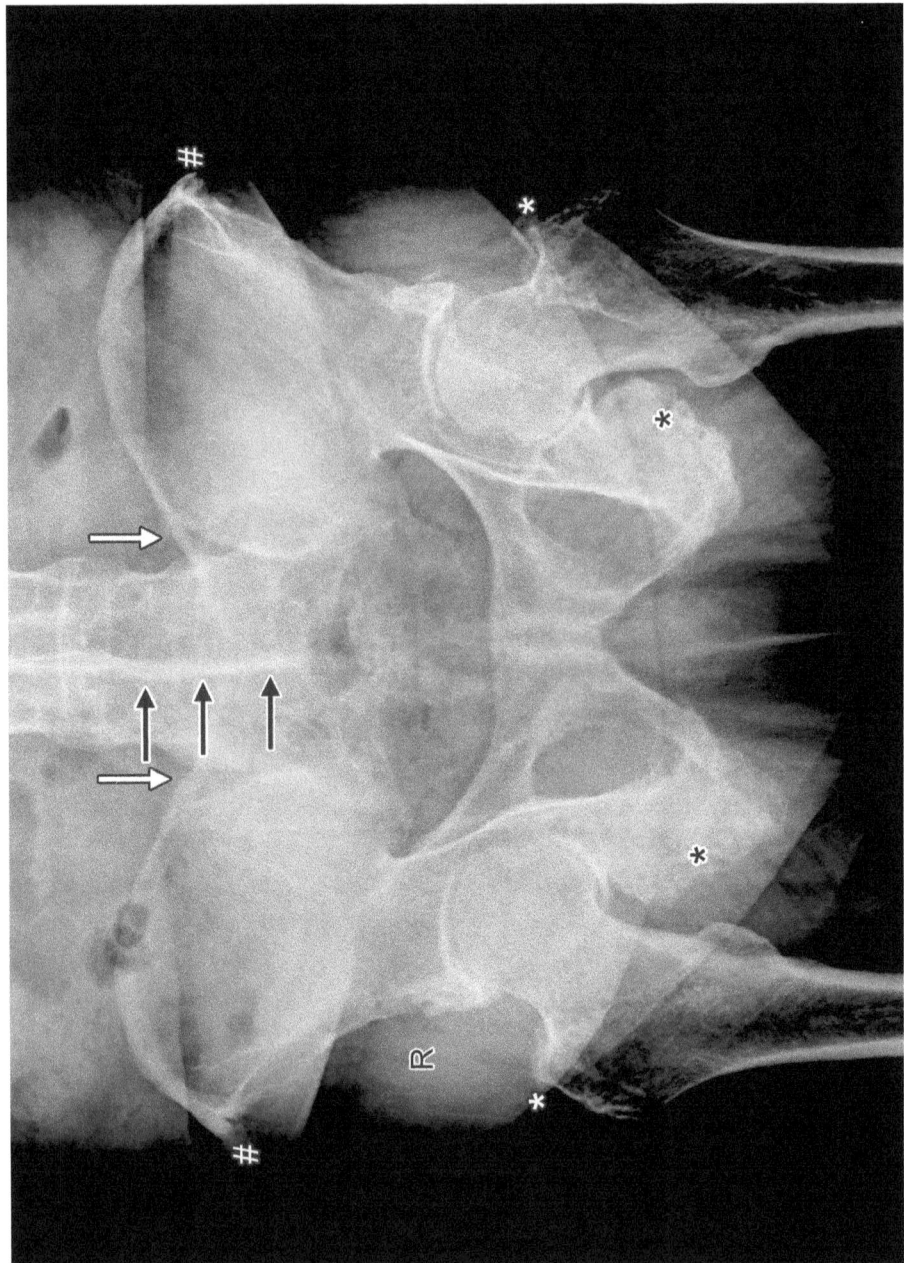

Fig. 12: Radiograph of pelvis, anteroposterior projection showing bilateral grade-4 sacroiliitis with Dagger sign (black arrows) due to the calcification of supraspinous ligament; proliferative changes and irregularity over both ischial tuberosities (black asterisks) and greater trochanters (white asterisks) suggestive of chronic enthesitis; enthesophytes (bony outgrowths) at both anterior superior iliac spines (hash) and calcification of bilateral iliolumbar ligaments (white arrows).

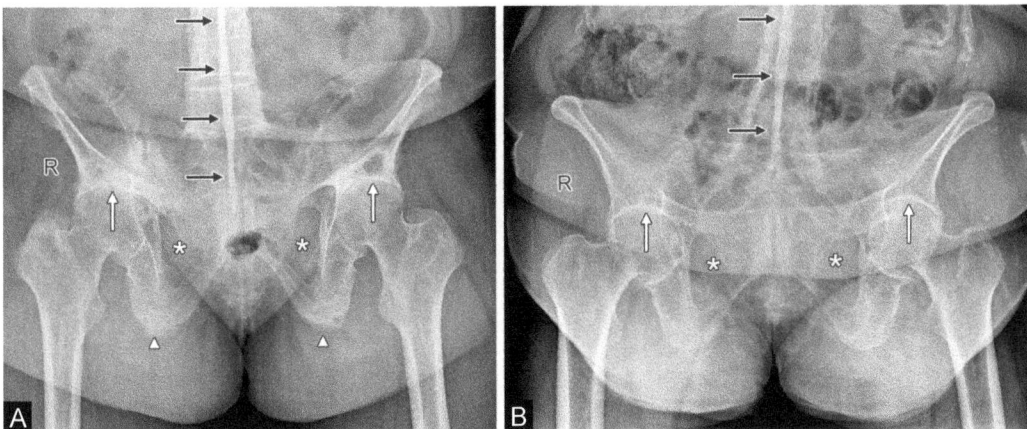

Figs. 13A and B: Radiographs of pelvis, anteroposterior projection of two patients with advanced, long-standing AS. Both the radiographs show Dagger sign (black arrows), reduced joint space in both hip joints (white arrows) and apparently large obturator foramina (white asterisks) due to the peculiar upward rotation of the pelvis, which is commonly seen in patients with advanced AS secondary to kyphotic deformity of the spine. Note is made of bony irregularity over both ischial tuberosities in image A (white arrowheads), suggestive of chronic enthesitis.

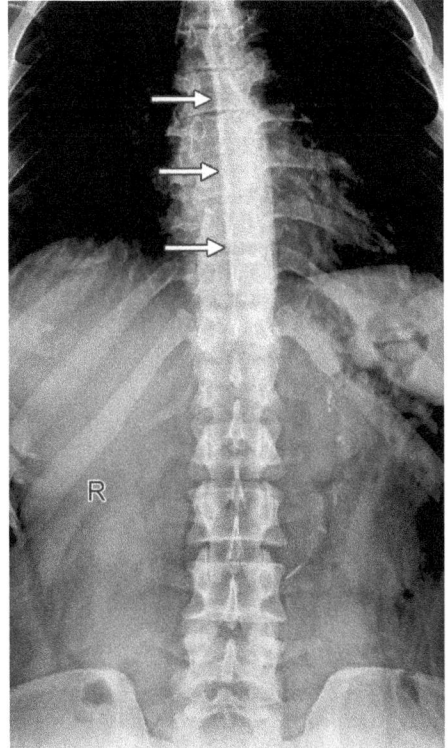

Fig. 14: Radiograph of thoracolumbar spine, anteroposterior projection showing a continuous straight line through the spinous processes of thoracic vertebrae which resembles Dagger sign (white arrows). However, this is a normal finding due to the overlap of spinous processes of thoracic vertebrae because of the normal kyphotic shape of the thoracic spine and should not be mistaken for Dagger sign.

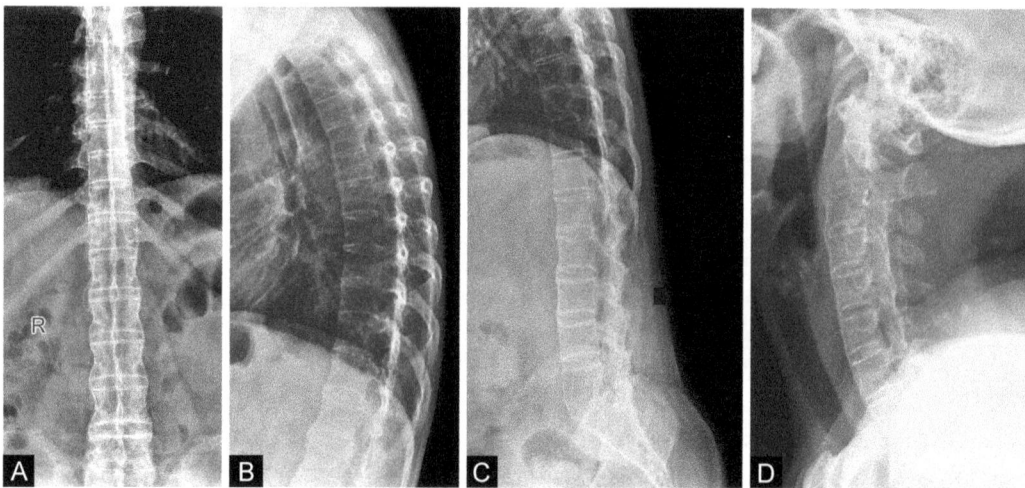

Figs. 15A to D: Radiographs of the spine showing calcification of annulus fibrosus of all the intervertebral discs in thoracic (A and B), lumbar (C) and cervical (D) spine. The appearance is called 'bamboo' spine in anteroposterior projection (A) due to the resemblance with bamboo stem. In addition, there is loss of the normal lordotic curvature of the cervical and lumbar spines with squaring of the vertebral bodies.

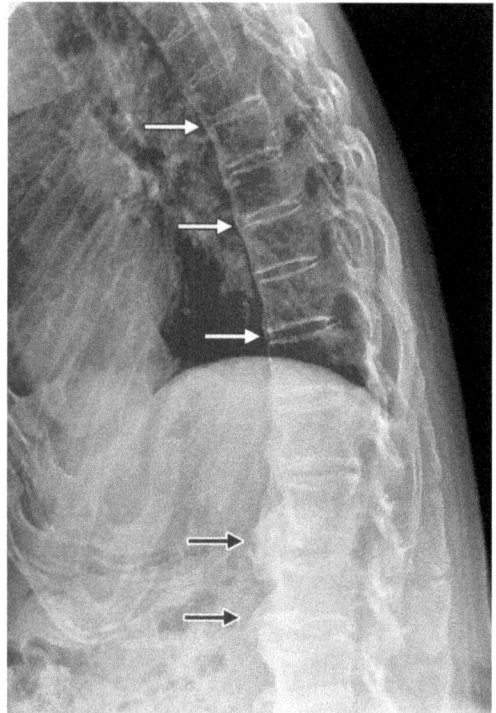

Fig. 16: Radiograph of thoracolumbar spine, lateral projection showing bulky osteophytes in the lumbar spine suggestive of degenerative changes (black arrows). Thoracic spine shows characteristic bridging syndesmophytes (white arrows). Diagnosis of SpA can be missed in such cases if thoracic spine is not imaged. This illustrates that thoracic spine shows prominent changes associated with SpA and therefore, should be imaged during the evaluation of patients with SpA.

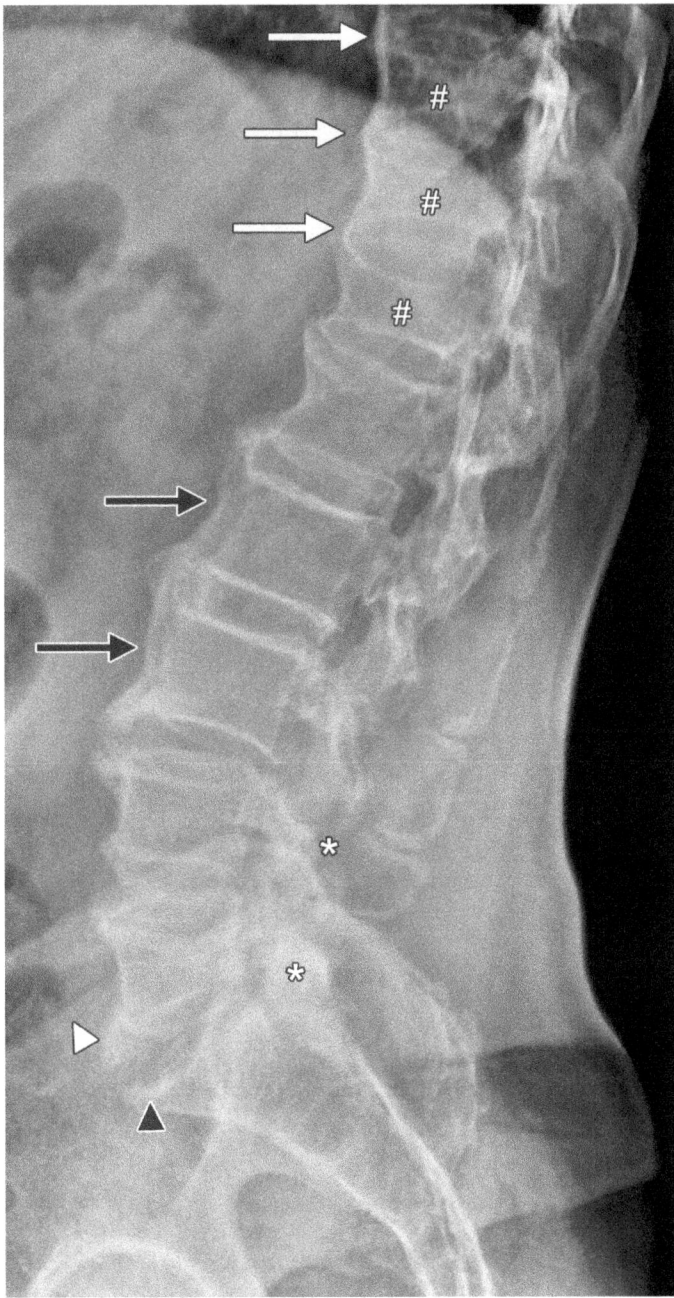

Fig. 17: Radiograph of lower thoracic and lumbar spine, lateral projection showing degenerative changes in the lumbar spine in the form of osteophytes (white arrowhead) and end-plate damage (black arrowhead), ossification of the anterior longitudinal ligament (black arrows) and sclerosis of facet joints, suggestive of facet joint arthropathy (white asterisks). Lower thoracic spine shows bridging syndesmophytes (white arrows) and morphometric compression fractures of the vertebral bodies (hash) characterized by flattened, 'biconcave' appearing vertebral bodies.

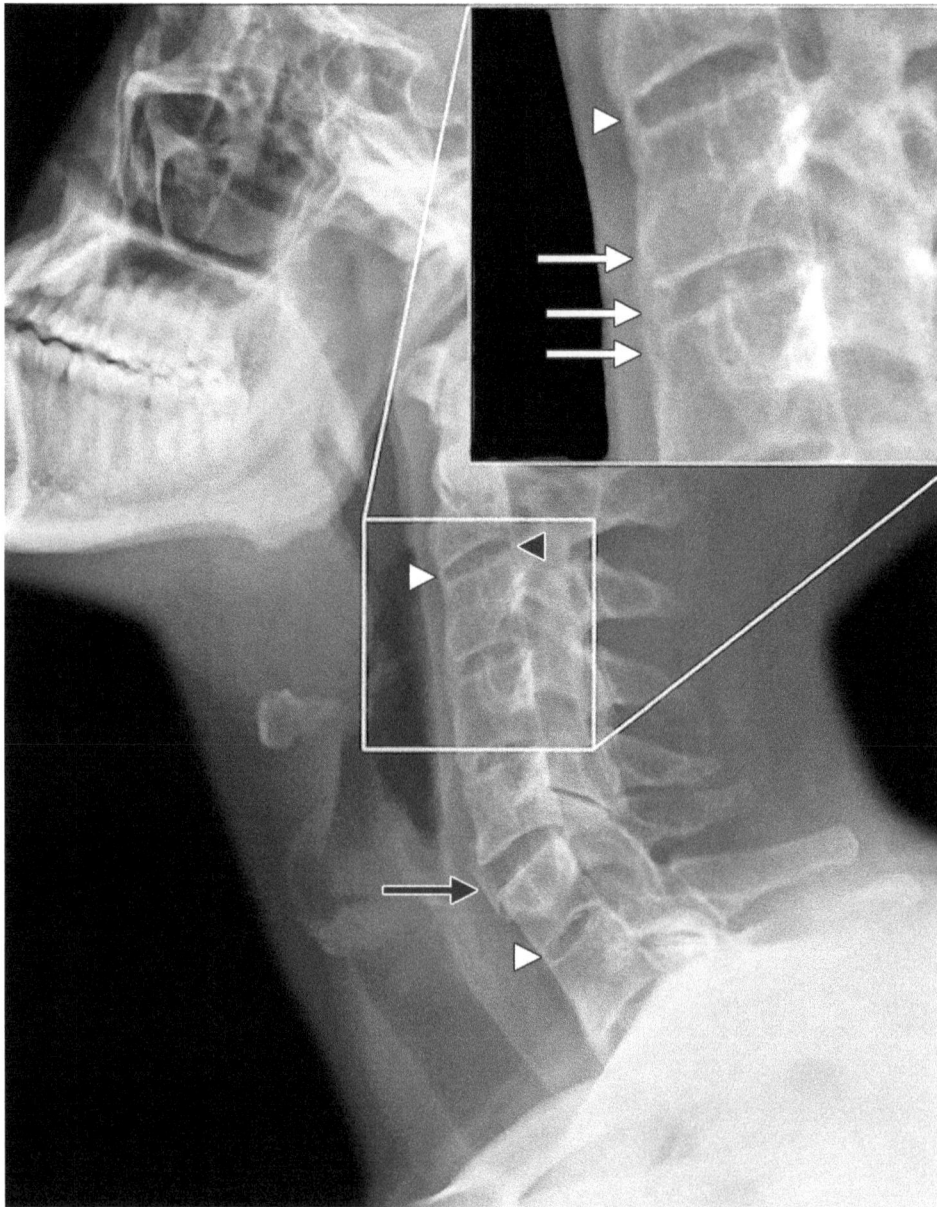

Fig. 18: Radiograph of cervical spine, lateral projection of a young male patient with AS showing both syndesmophytes and ossification of anterior longitudinal ligament (OALL). White arrowheads show thin areas of linear calcification along the annulus fibrosus, in line with the anterior borders of the vertebrae—these are syndesmophytes. Similar lesions are seen posteriorly (black arrowhead). Black arrow shows a thick area of calcification, anterior to the alignment of vertebral bodies, suggestive of patchy OALL. Similarly, areas marked by white arrows in the zoomed inset show patchy areas of calcification which extend beyond the limits of annulus fibrosus and attached at the ends of the anterior borders of vertebral bodies above and below, suggestive of patchy OALL (white arrows), and not syndesmophytes (marked by white arrowhead in the zoomed inset).

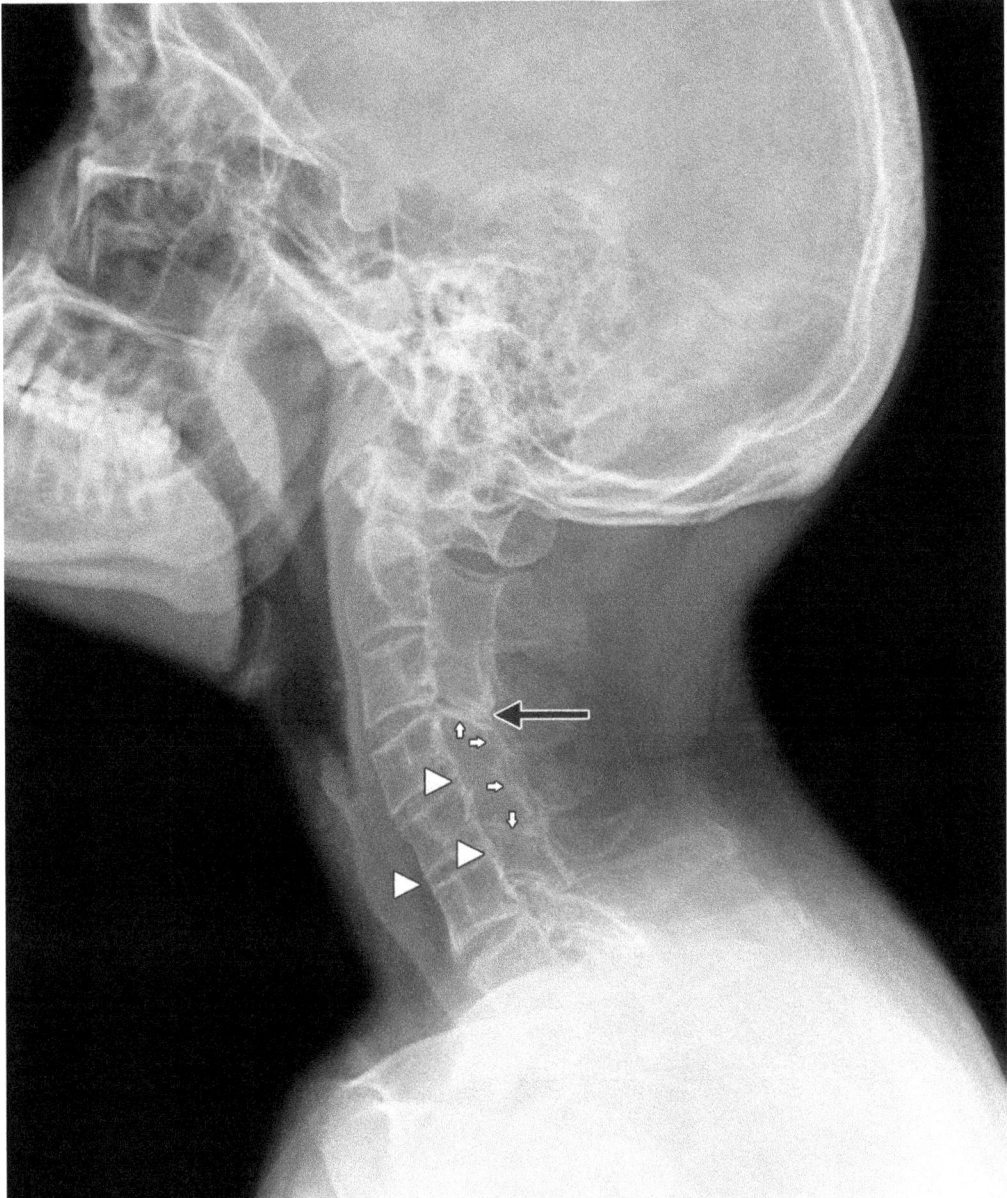

Fig. 19: Radiograph of cervical spine, lateral projection, showing anterior and posterior bridging syndesmophytes (white arrowheads) and calcification of ligamentum flavum (borders marked by white arrows) with sclerosis of a facet joint (black arrow).

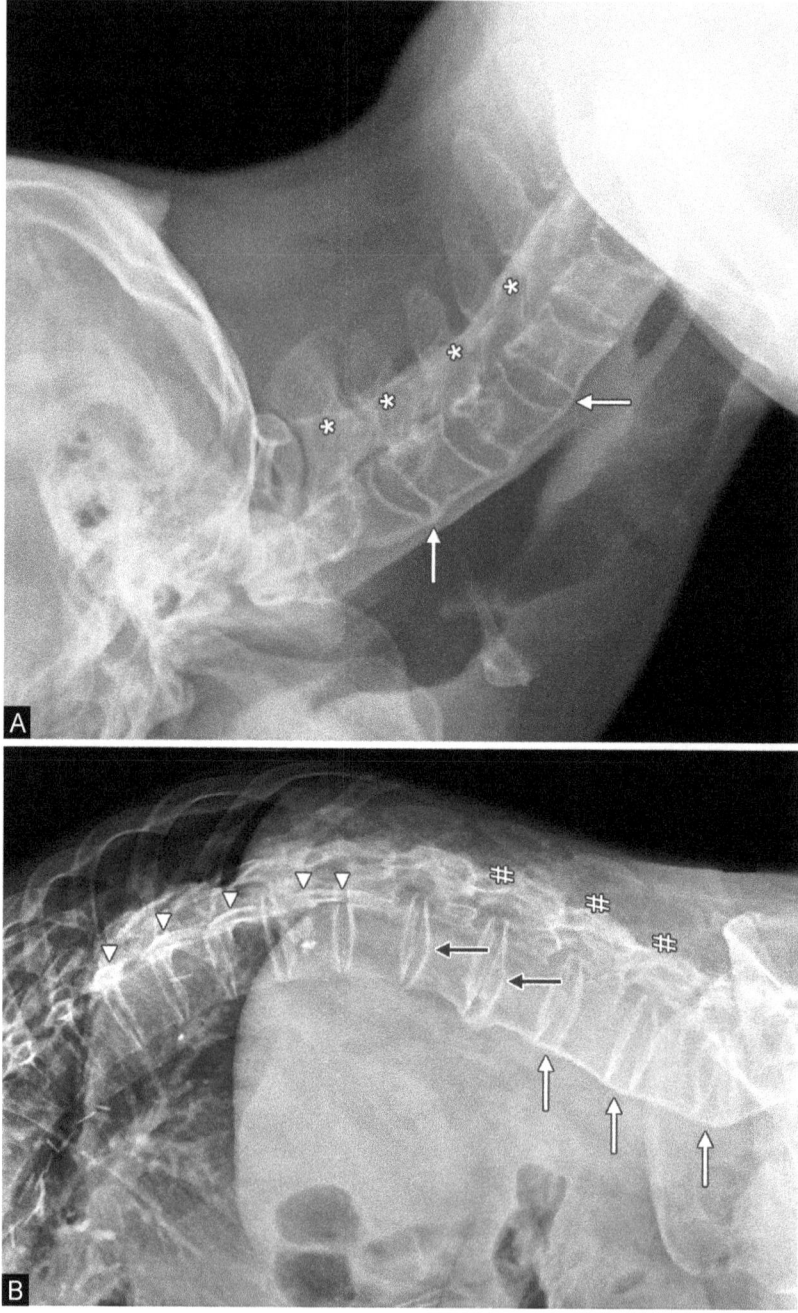

Figs. 20A and B: (A) Radiograph of the cervical spine of a patient with long-standing advanced AS showing multiple bridging anterior syndesmophytes (white arrows) and extensive calcification of the ligamentum flavum (white asterisks); (B) Radiograph of the thoracolumbar spine of the same patient showing multiple bridging syndesmophytes (white arrows); severely osteoporotic square-shaped appearance of the vertebral bodies; kyphosis; sclerosis of the facet joints (hash) and ossification of posterior longitudinal ligament (white arrowheads); indentation of the superior endplates of L2 and L3, suggestive of morphometric fractures (black arrows).

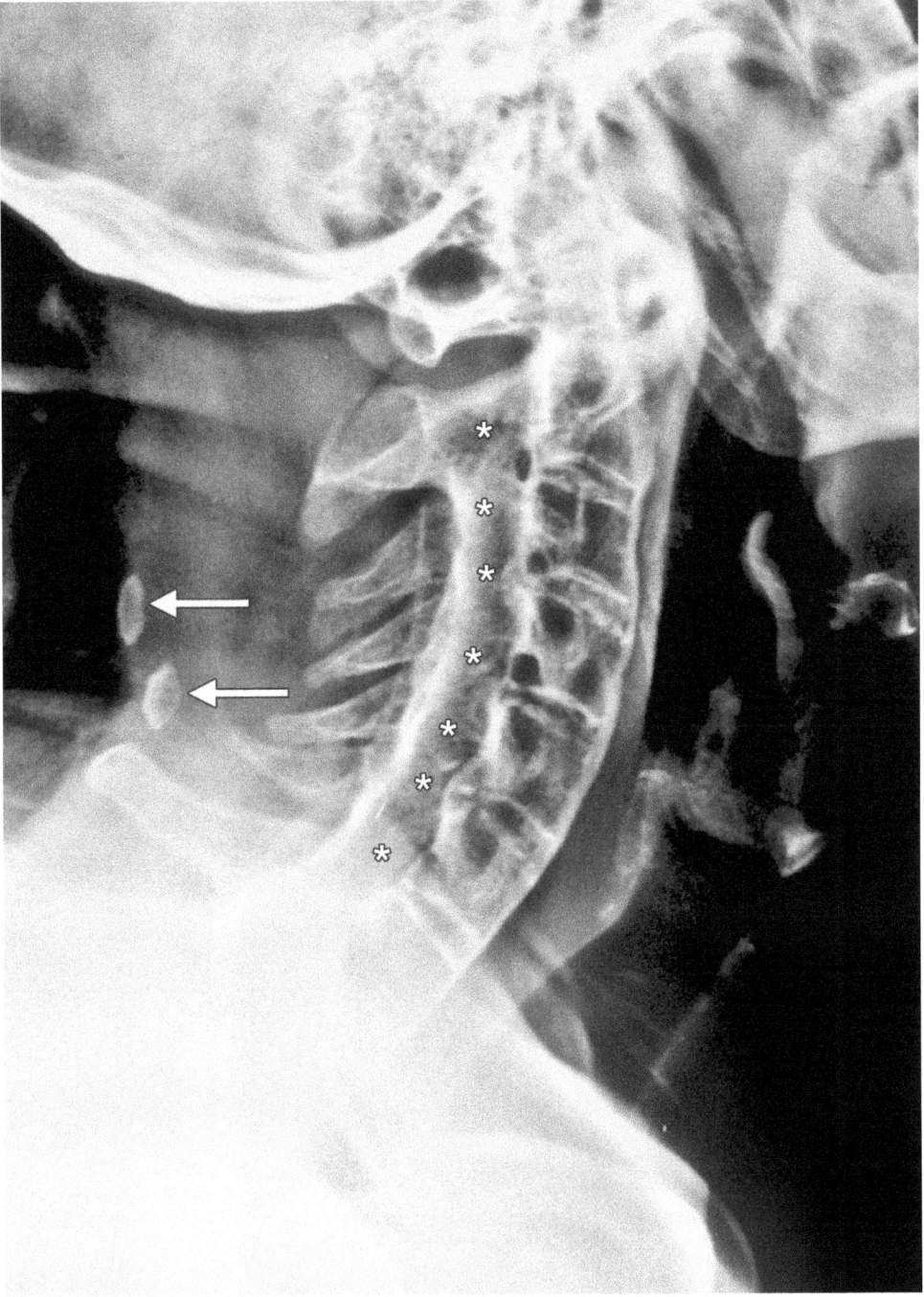

Fig. 21: Radiograph of cervical spine, lateral projection showing multiple bridging syndesmophytes. Calcification of ligamentum flavum (asterisks) and ligamentum nuchae is observed (white arrows).

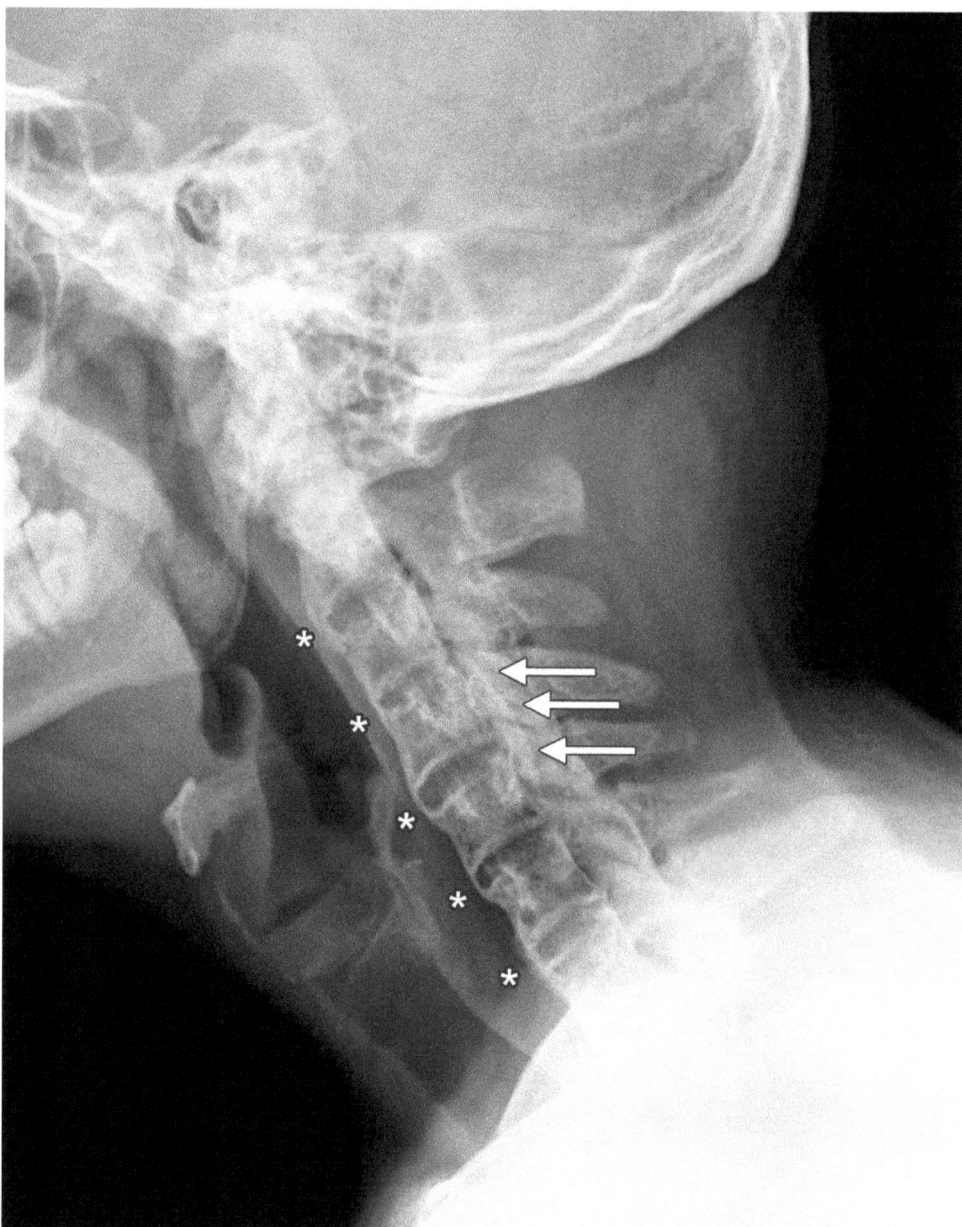

Fig. 22: Radiograph of cervical spine, lateral projection showing multiple bridging syndesmophytes (asterisks) and ossification of posterior longitudinal ligament (white arrows). Note is also made of ligamentum flavum calcification.

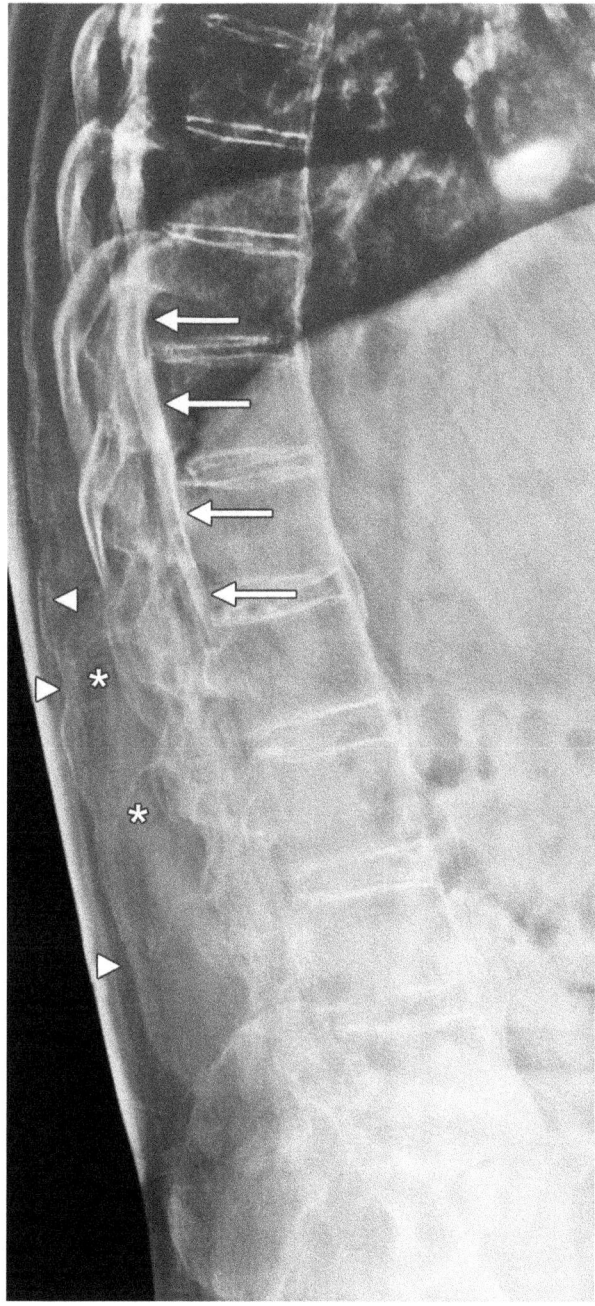

Fig. 23: Radiograph of thoracolumbar spine, lateral projection showing multiple bridging syndesmophytes. Ossification of posterior longitudinal ligament (arrows), supraspinous ligament (arrowheads) and interspinous ligaments (obliteration of the space between the spinous processes [asterisks]) is also seen.

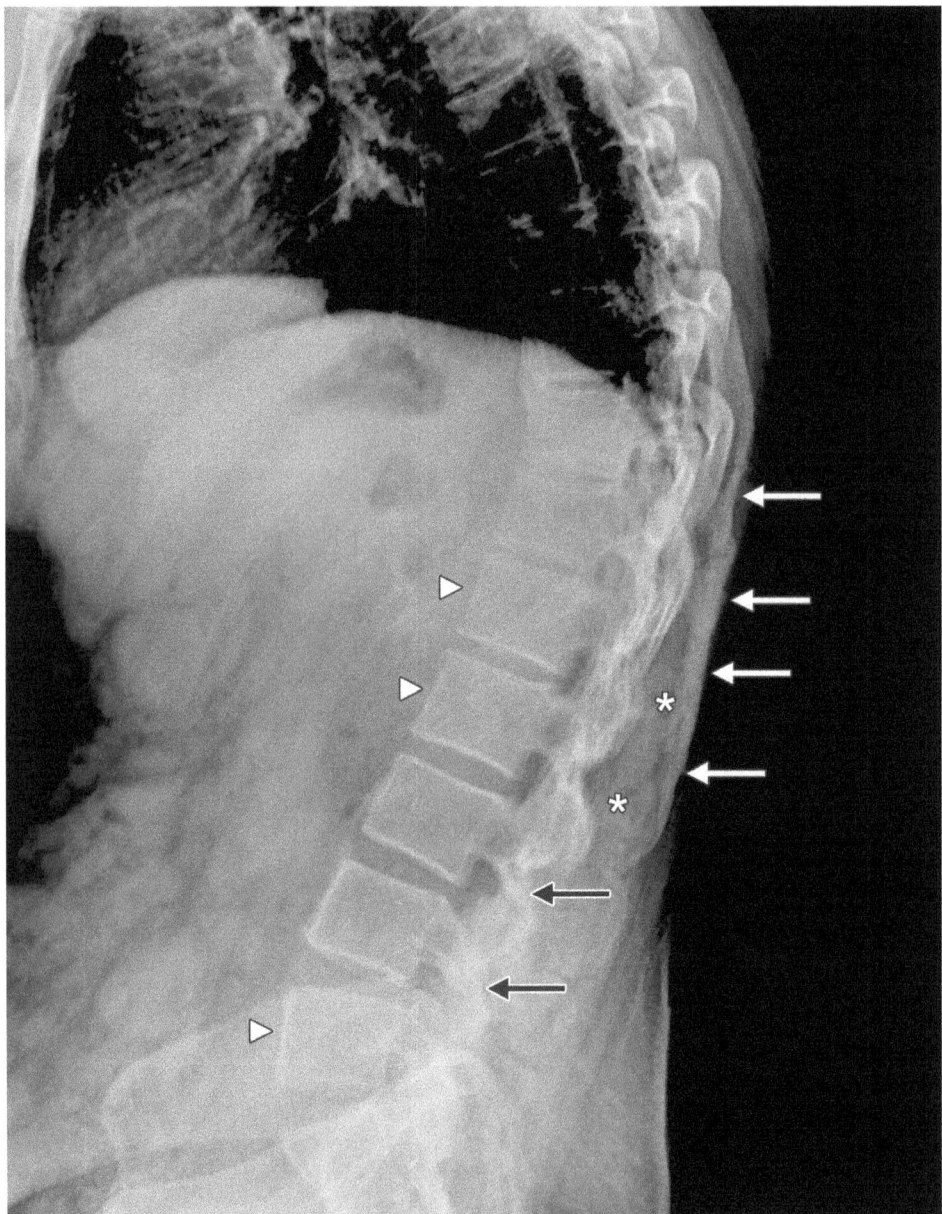

Fig. 24: Radiograph of thoracolumbar spine, lateral projection showing loss of anterior concavity of vertebral bodies giving rise to the appearance of 'squaring' (white arrowheads); ossification of the supraspinous ligament (white arrows); obliteration of the space between spinous processes of the upper lumbar vertebrae due to calcification of interspinous ligament (asterisks); and facet joint sclerosis (black arrows).

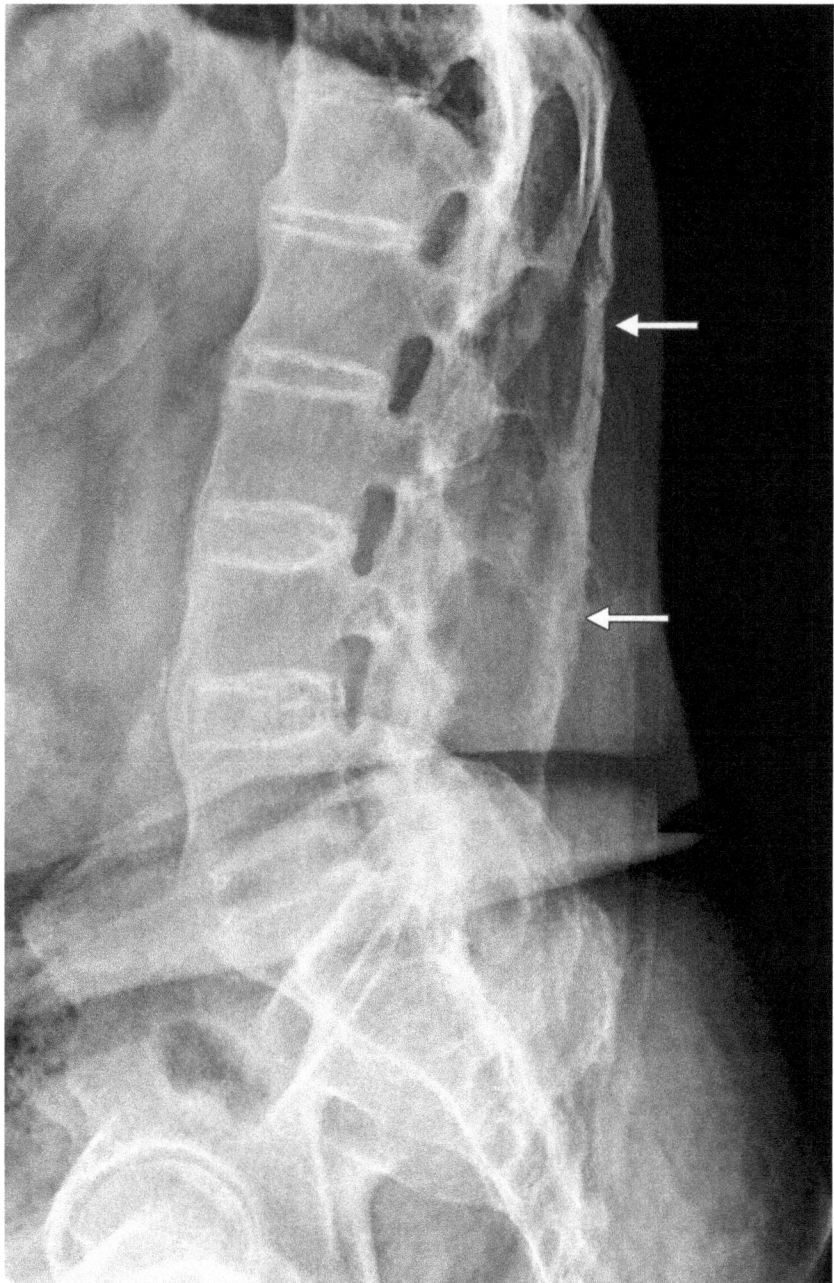

Fig. 25: Radiograph of lumbar spine, lateral projection showing multiple bridging syndesmophytes with ossification of supraspinous (arrows) ligament.

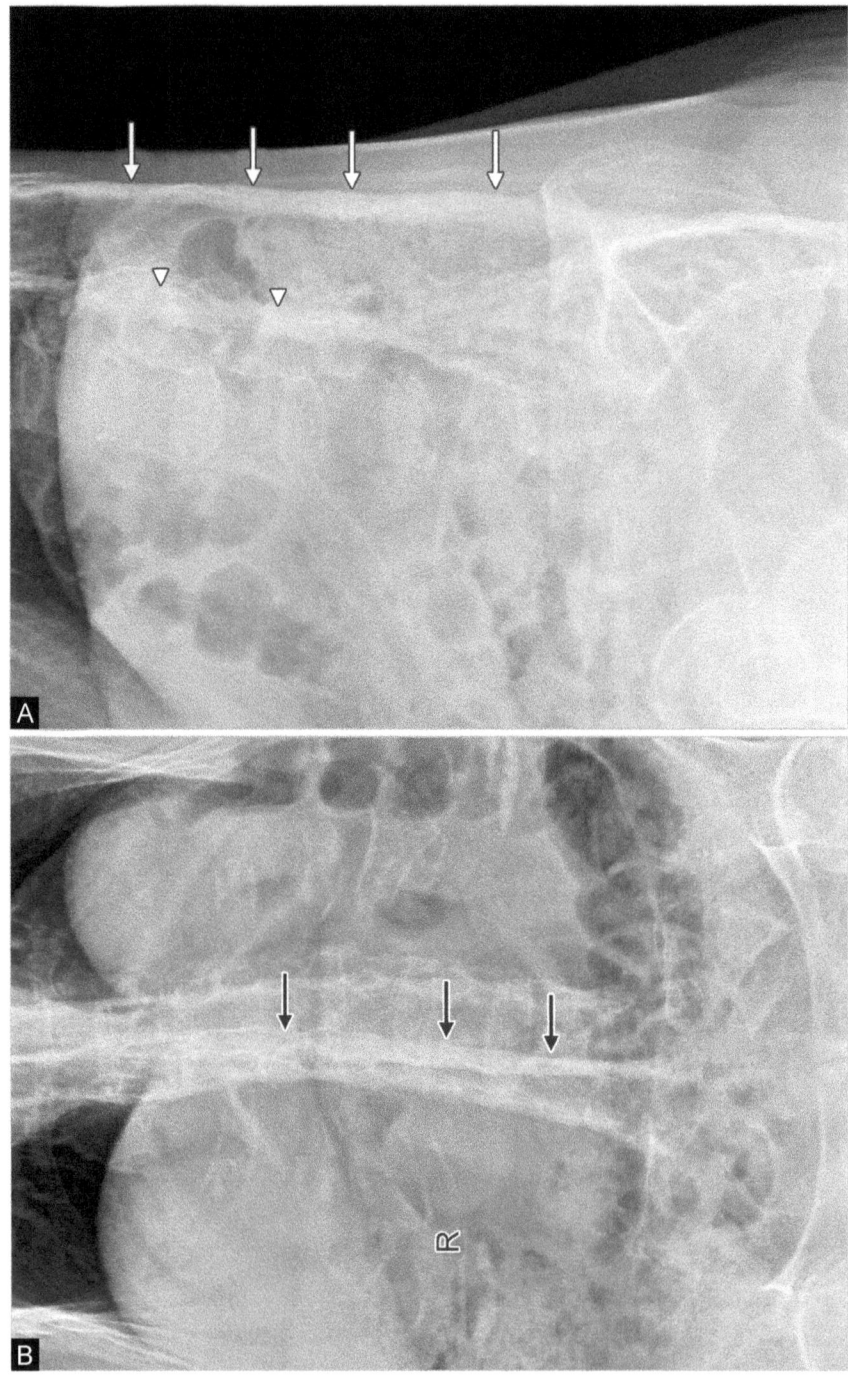

Figs. 26A and B: Radiograph of lower thoracic and lumbar spine showing calcification of the supraspinous ligament in lateral projection (white arrows in A) giving rise to Dagger sign visible in anteroposterior projection (black arrows in B). Note is made of sclerosis of facet joints (white arrowheads in A).

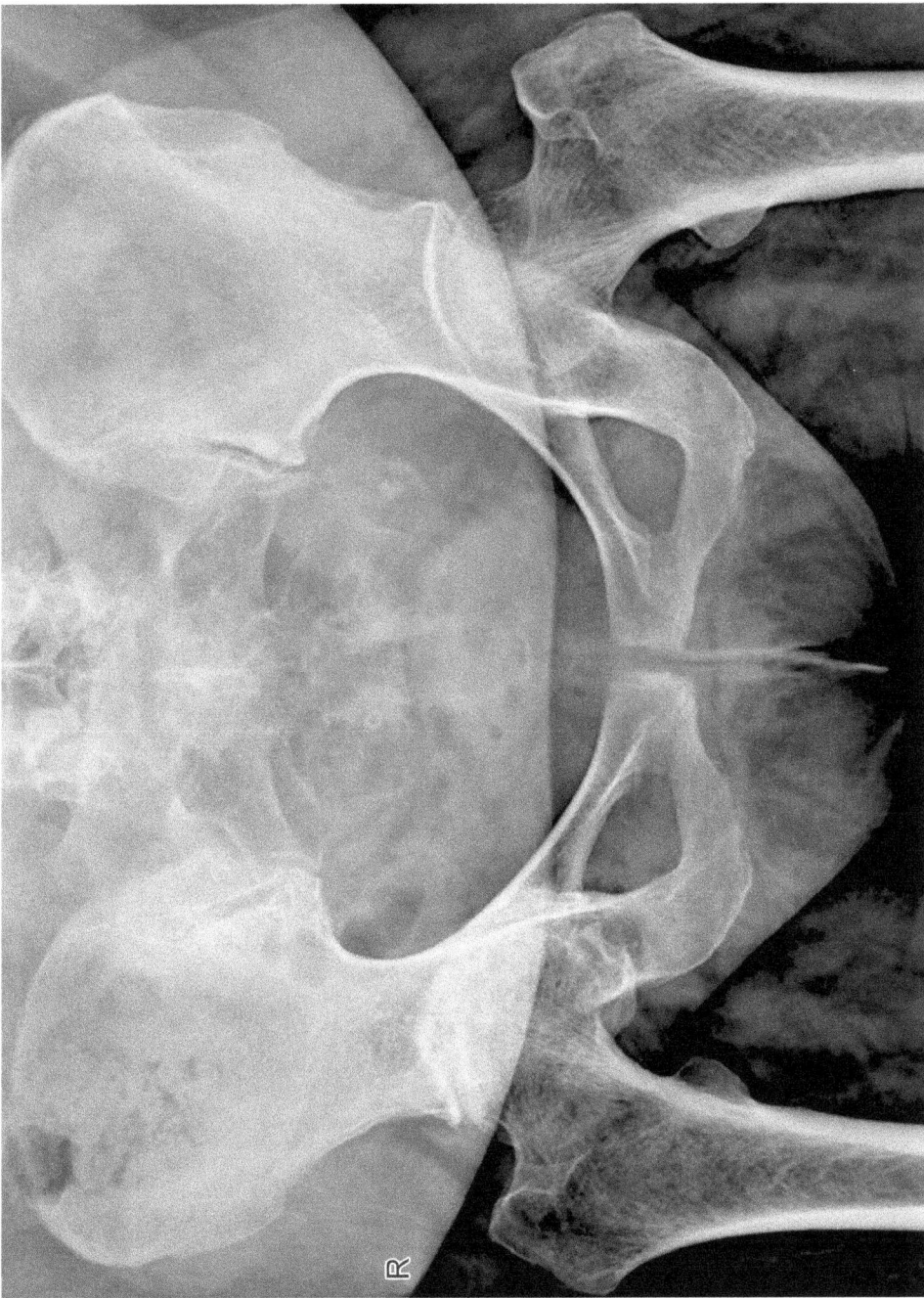

Fig. 27: Radiograph of the pelvis anteroposterior view of a 42-year old lady with peripheral SpA showing damaged right hip joint—uniform joint space reduction, subarticular sclerosis and cysts.

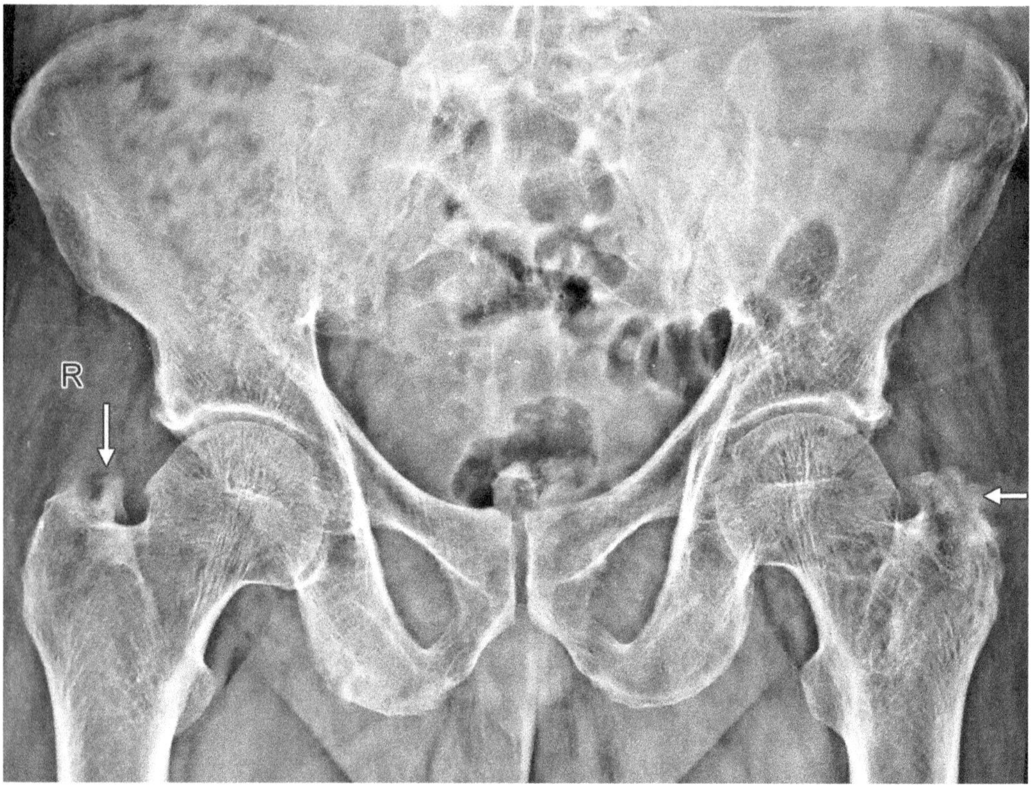

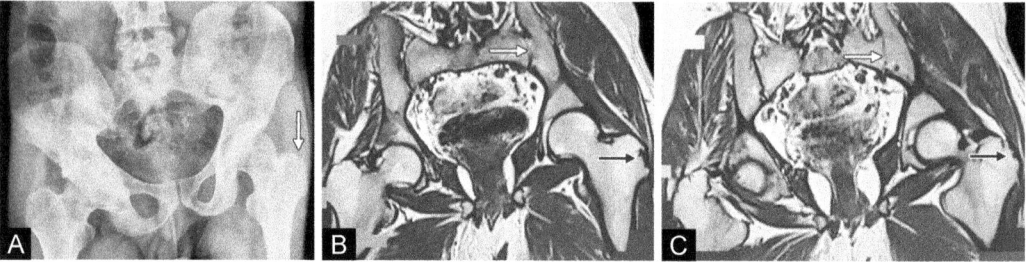

Fig. 28: Radiograph of pelvis, anteroposterior projection of a patient with advanced AS showing bony outgrowths (enthesophytes) at both greater trochanters (arrows), suggestive of chronic enthesitis.

Figs. 29A to C: (A) Radiograph of pelvis, anteroposterior projection showing irregularity of left greater trochanter (white arrow), suggestive of chronic enthesitis. (B and C) MRI of pelvis of the same patient (coronal view, T1W sequence) showing erosions in the left greater trochanter (black arrows), confirming the presence of chronic enthesopathy. Note is also made of right grade-3 and left grade-4 sacroiliitis in image A. Partial ankylosis of left SIJ is noted on MRI in B and C (white arrows).

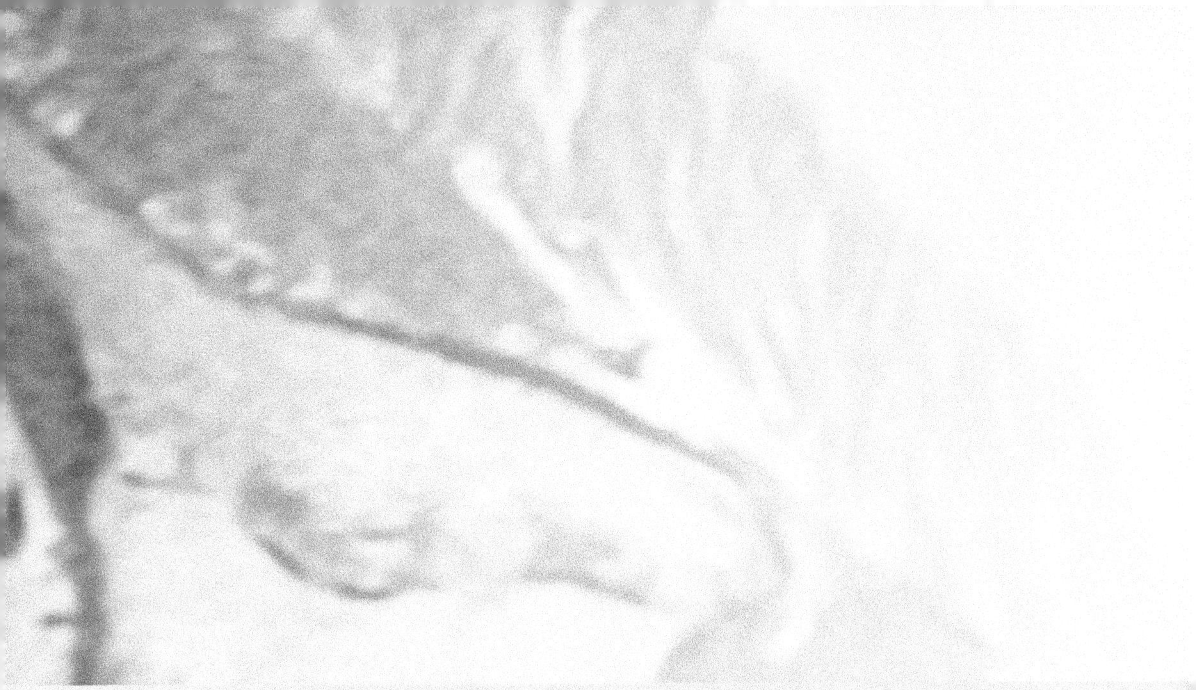

MRI OF SACROILIAC JOINT

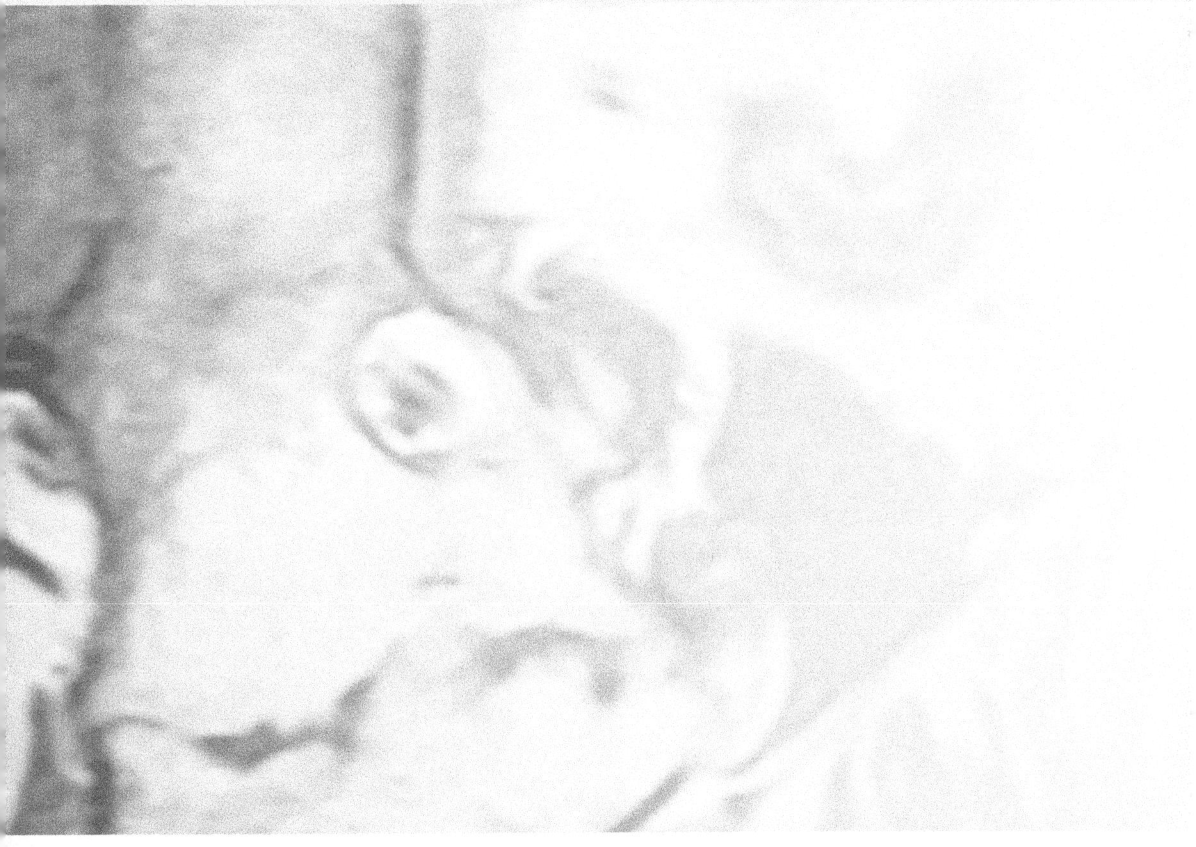

32 | A Rheumatologist's Guide to Interpreting Imaging in Spondyloarthritis

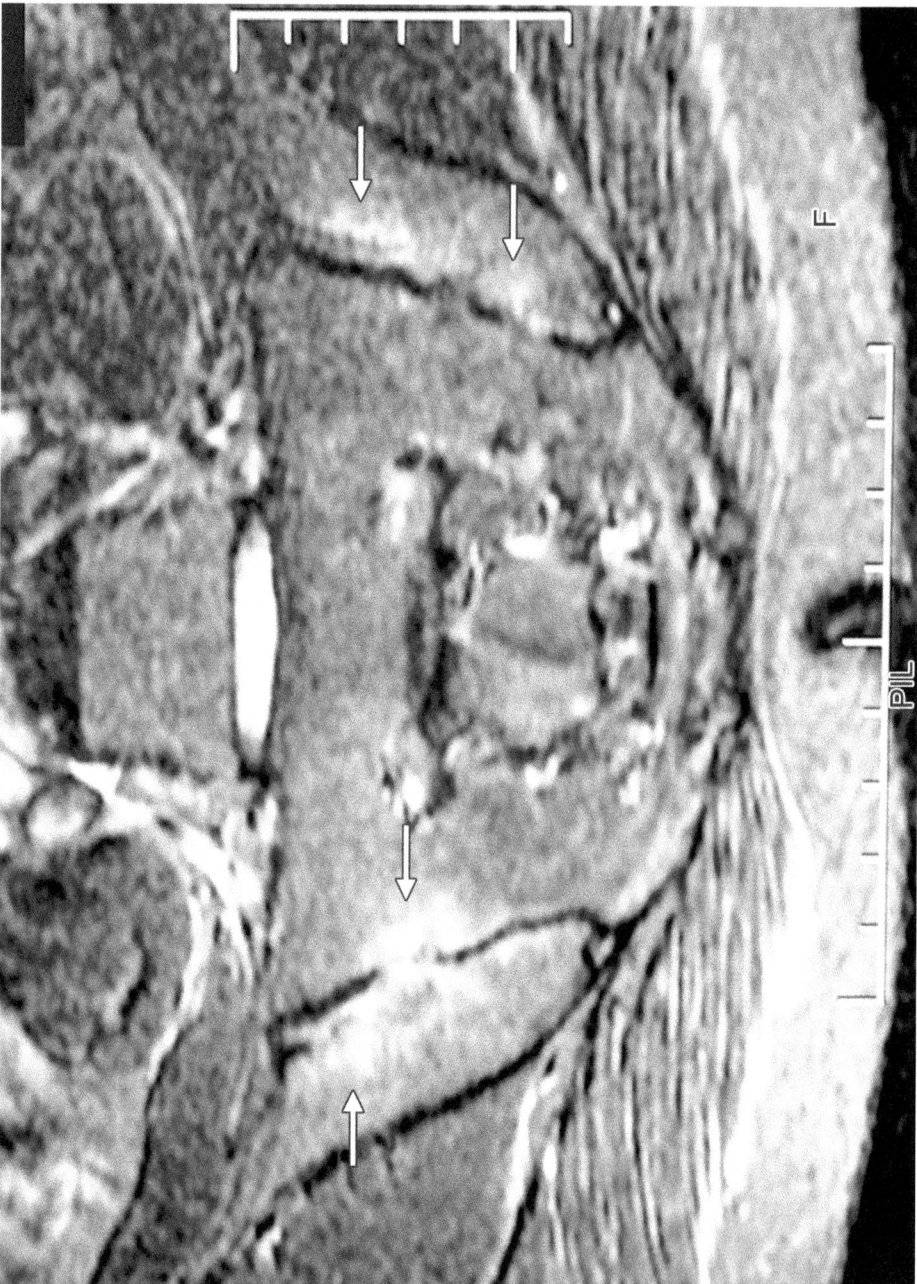

Fig. 30: MRI of sacroiliac joint (SIJ) short tau inversion recovery (STIR) sequence (bright intervertebral disc and dark subcutaneous fat [F]) showing bright signal in the subarticular portions of both SIJ (white arrows), suggestive of bone marrow edema.

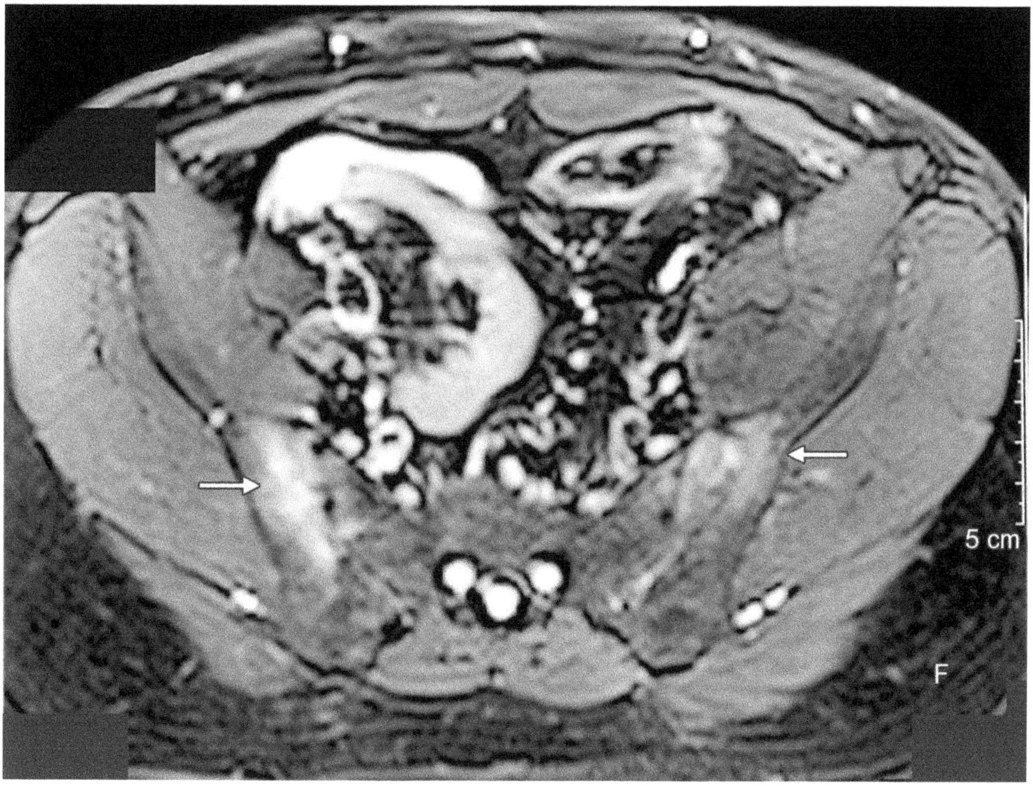

MRI of Sacroiliac Joint

Fig. 31: MRI of SIJ, axial section, STIR sequence (dark subcutaneous fat [F]) showing periarticular bright signal intensity in both SIJ, suggestive of bone marrow edema (arrows).

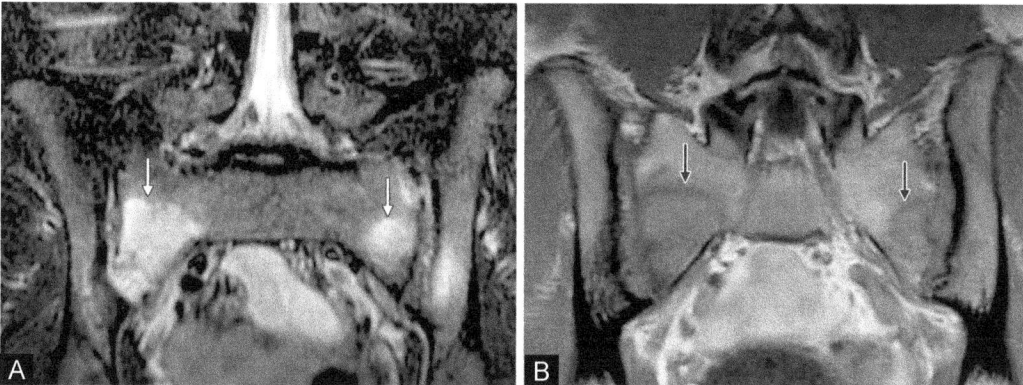

Figs. 32A and B: Coronal section of MRI of SIJ showing bright signal intensity along both SIJ on STIR sequence (white arrows in A) and dark signal intensities in corresponding areas on T1 sequence (black arrows in B), suggestive of bone marrow edema.

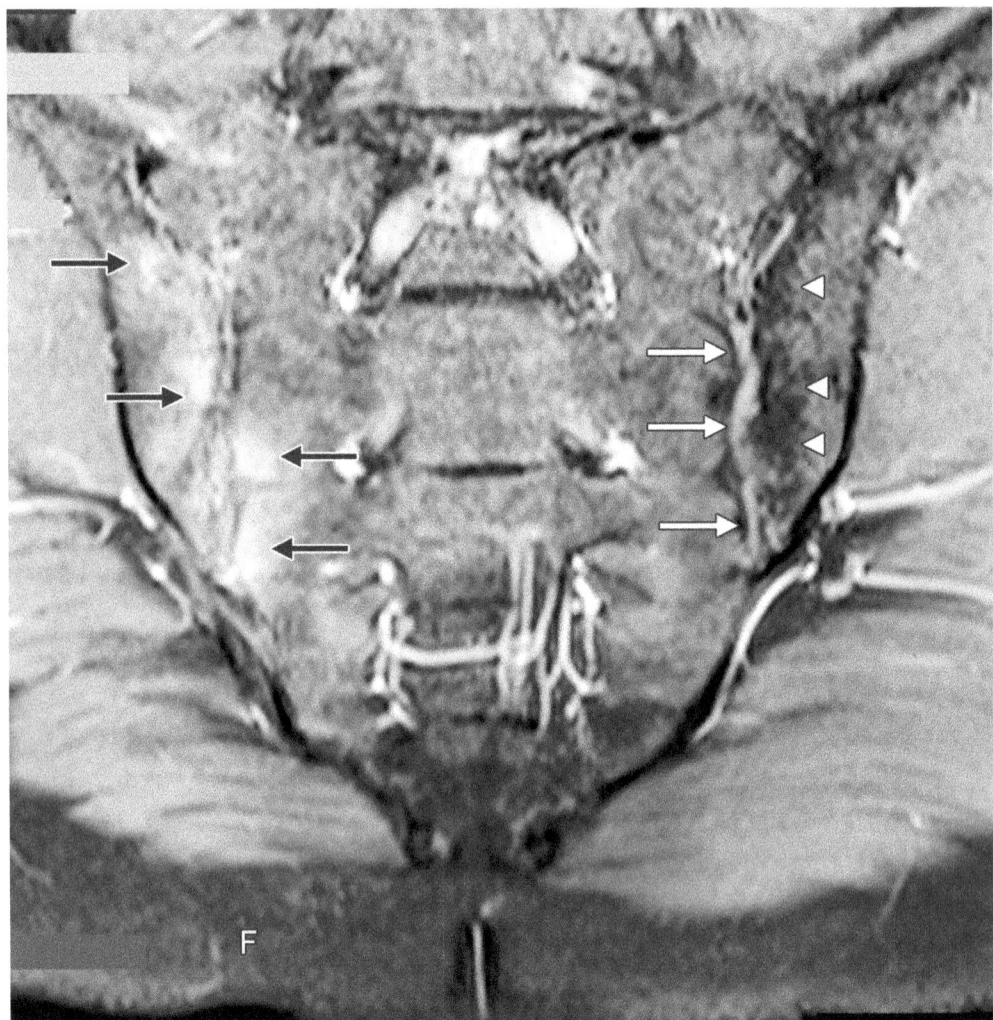

Fig. 33: Coronal section of MRI of SIJ STIR sequence (dark subcutaneous fat [F]) showing bright signal intensity in periarticular areas of right SIJ suggestive of bone marrow edema (black arrows); dark signal along the iliac aspect of left SIJ, suggestive of sclerosis (white arrowheads) and bright signal intensity in the left sacroiliac joint cavity suggestive of synovitis (white arrows).

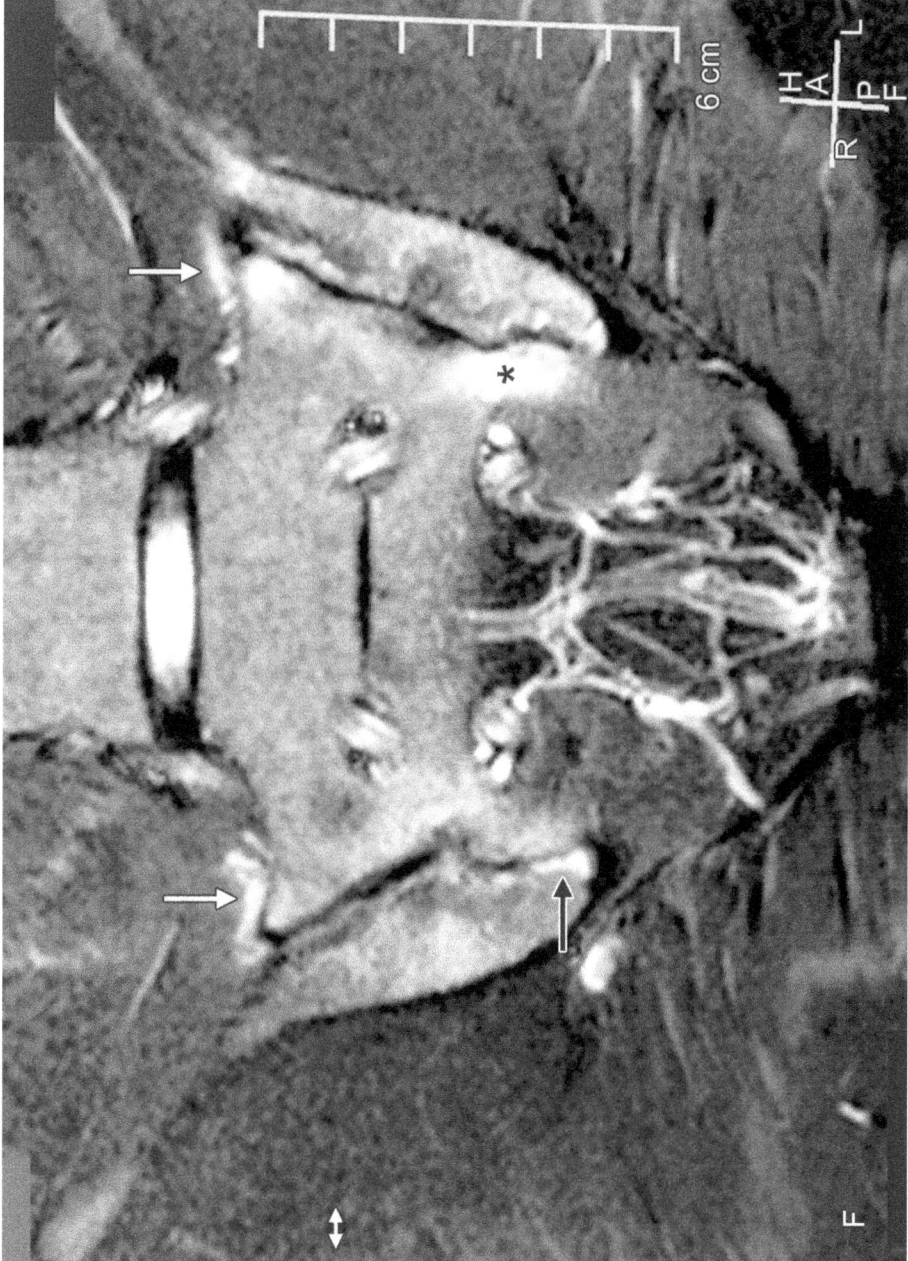

Fig. 34: MRI of SIJ, coronal STIR image (bright intervertebral disc and dark subcutaneous fat [F]) showing subarticular bone marrow edema in left SIJ (asterisk); bright signals at the superior edge of both SIJ (white arrows), suggestive of capsulitis; bright signal in the synovial cavity of lowest part of right SIJ, suggestive of synovitis (black arrow).

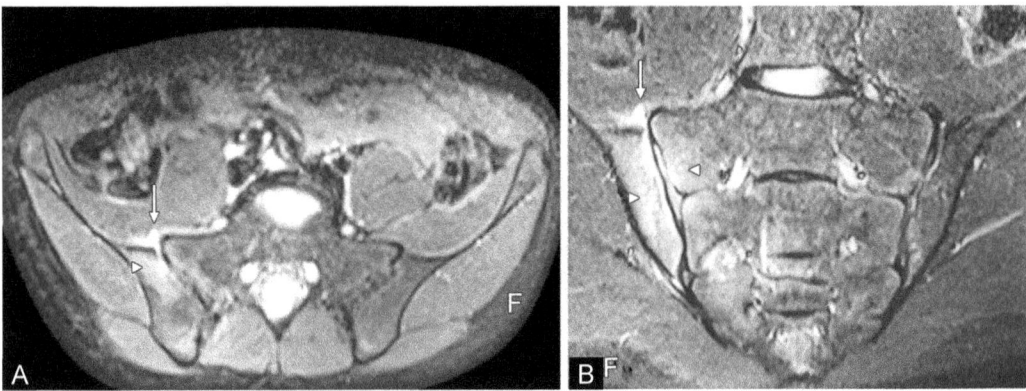

Figs. 35A and B: MRI of SIJ, STIR sequences (dark subcutaneous fat in A and B [F] and bright intervertebral disc in B) of the same patient showing capsulitis (white arrows) and bone marrow edema (arrowheads) in the right SIJ in the axial section (A) and coronal section (B).

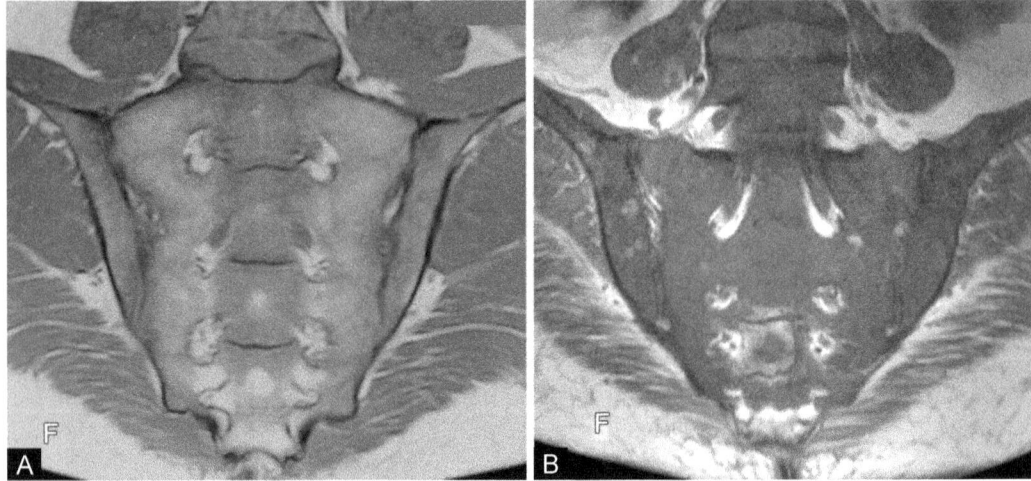

Figs. 36A and B: (A) Coronal section of T1W MRI (dark intervertebral disc and bright subcutaneous fat [F]) of SIJ of a 62-year old male showing normal SIJ and normal fatty appearance of sacrum and ilium due to the presence of bone marrow fat; (B) Coronal section of T1W MRI of a 60-year old male suffering from chronic myeloid leukemia. Note the loss of bright fatty signals in the sacrum and ilium due to the replacement of bone marrow fat with neoplastic hematopoietic cells.

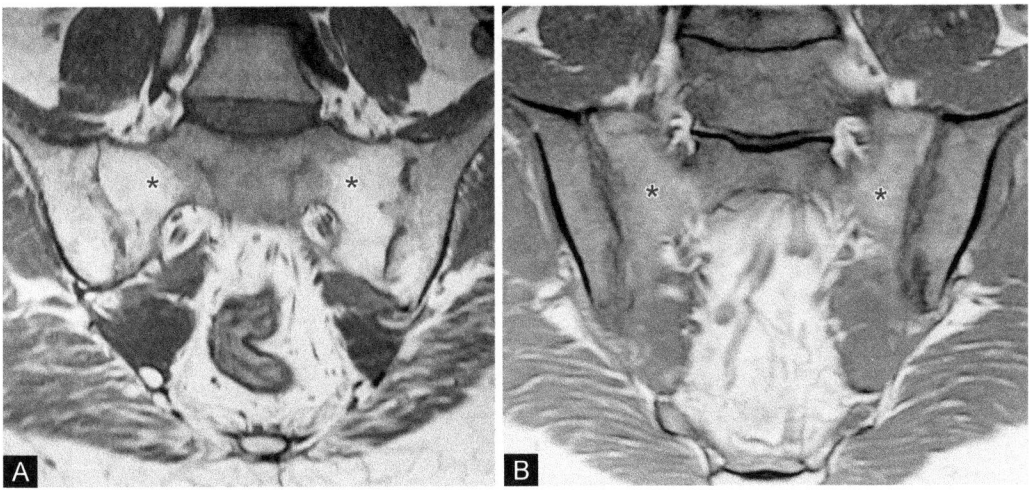

Figs. 37A and B: MRI of SIJ, coronal sections, T1W sequences differentiating fatty metaplasia from normal bone marrow fatty signal. (A) intense, homogeneous, sharply demarcated bright signal intensities in the subarticular areas of both SIJ (black asterisks), suggestive of fatty metaplasia; (B) Bright signal intensities in the subarticular areas are heterogeneous and have poorly demarcated borders (black asterisks), as compared to A. This is the appearance of normal fatty bone marrow signal.[6]

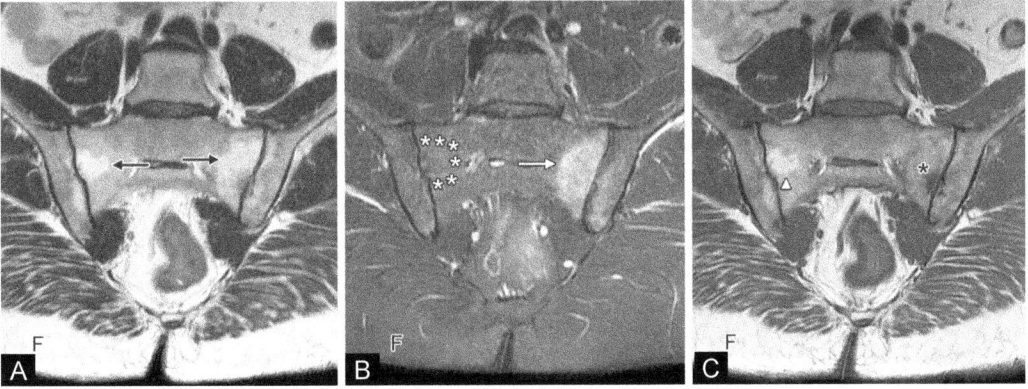

Figs. 38A to C: MRI of SIJ, coronal sections. (A) T2W sequence (bright intervertebral disc and subcutaneous fat [F]) showing bright signal intensities along both SIJ (black arrows). Since the sequence is not fat-suppressed, the lesions could be bone marrow edema or fatty metaplasia—the differentiation is difficult on this sequence alone; (B) STIR sequence (bright intervertebral disc and dark subcutaneous fat [F]) of the same patient with section at the same level as A, showing dark signal along right SIJ (surrounded by white asterisks, corresponding to the bright area in image A) and bright signal along left SIJ (white arrow, corresponding to the bright area in image A), suggesting that former is fatty metaplasia and latter is bone marrow edema; (C) T1W sequence (dark intervertebral disc and bright subcutaneous fat [F]) of the same patient with section at same level showing bright signal along the right SIJ (fatty metaplasia) (white arrowhead) and dark signal along left SIJ (bone marrow edema) (black asterisk).

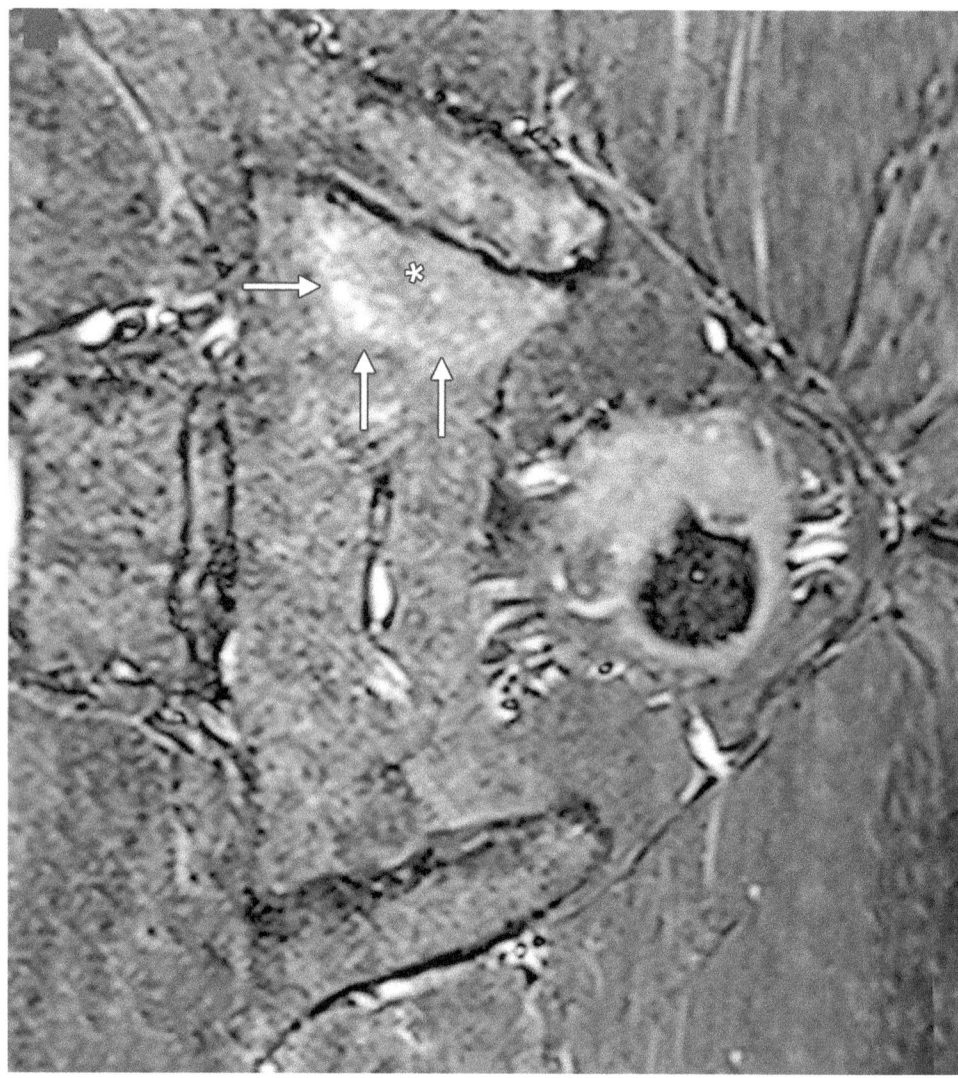

Fig. 39: MRI of SIJ, coronal section, STIR sequence showing bone marrow edema away from the joint line of left SIJ (white arrows) at the perimeter of a dark area (white asterisk). This appearance of 'rim bone marrow edema' is highly suggestive of SpA.

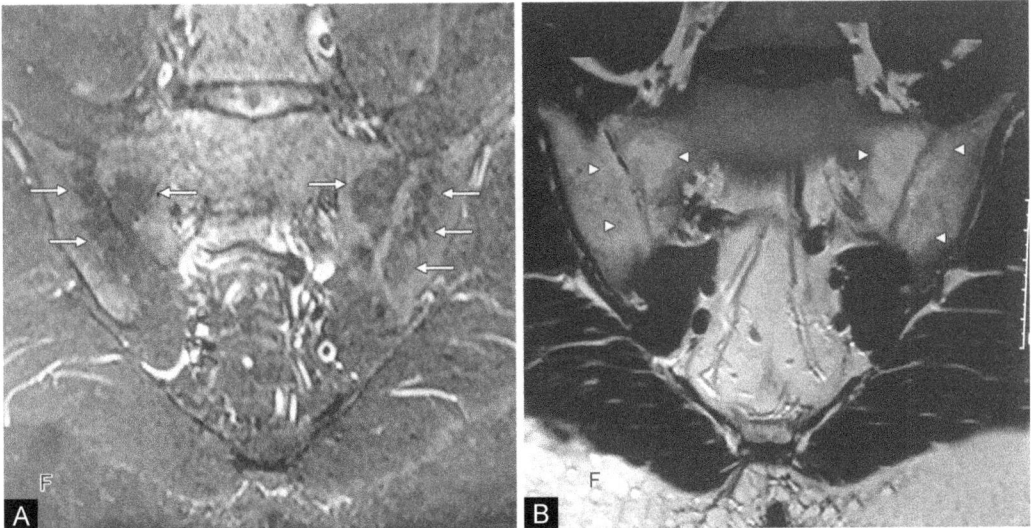

Figs. 40A and B: Coronal sections of the MRI of SIJ. (A) STIR sequence (bright intervertebral disc and dark subcutaneous fat [F]) showing dark signals along both SIJ (white arrows). This appearance on STIR can occur due to fatty metaplasia or sclerosis; (B) T1W sequence (dark intervertebral disc and bright subcutaneous fat [F]) of the same patient showing bright signals in the corresponding areas in A (white arrowheads), suggestive of fatty metaplasia. Sclerosis will give rise to dark signal on both STIR and T1W sequences.

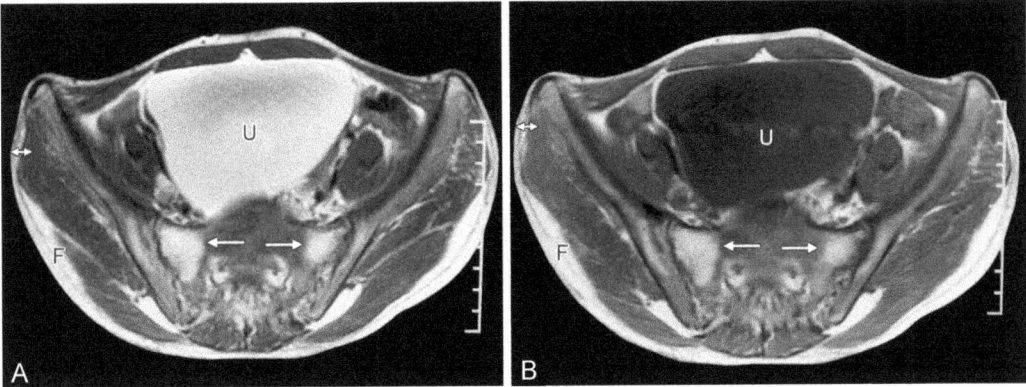

Figs. 41A and B: Axial sections of the MRI of SIJ. (A) T2W sequence (bright subcutaneous fat [F] and urine [U]) showing bright signals along both SIJ (white arrows). Since the sequence is not fat-suppressed, the lesions could be bone marrow edema or fatty metaplasia. (B) T1W sequence of the same patient (bright subcutaneous fat [F] and dark urine [U]) showing bright signals at the same location as in A. Bright signals on both T1 and T2 are suggestive of fatty metaplasia (bone marrow edema will appear bright on T2, STIR and contrast-enhanced T1 and dark on non-contrast T1).

40 A Rheumatologist's Guide to Interpreting Imaging in Spondyloarthritis

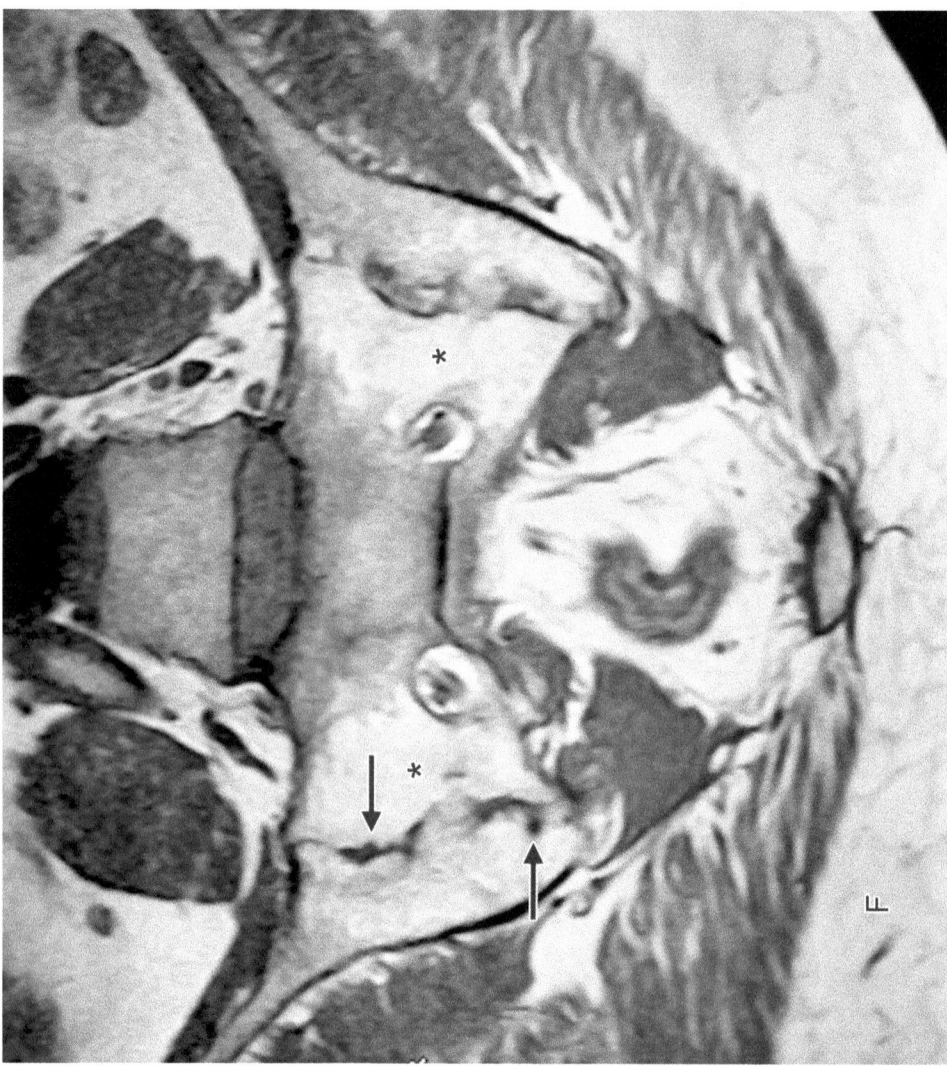

Fig. 42: Coronal T1W MRI of SIJ (dark intervertebral disc and bright subcutaneous fat [F]) showing bilateral bright signals, more along the sacral aspect of SIJ suggestive of fatty metaplasia (asterisks) with periarticular erosions in the right SIJ (black arrows).

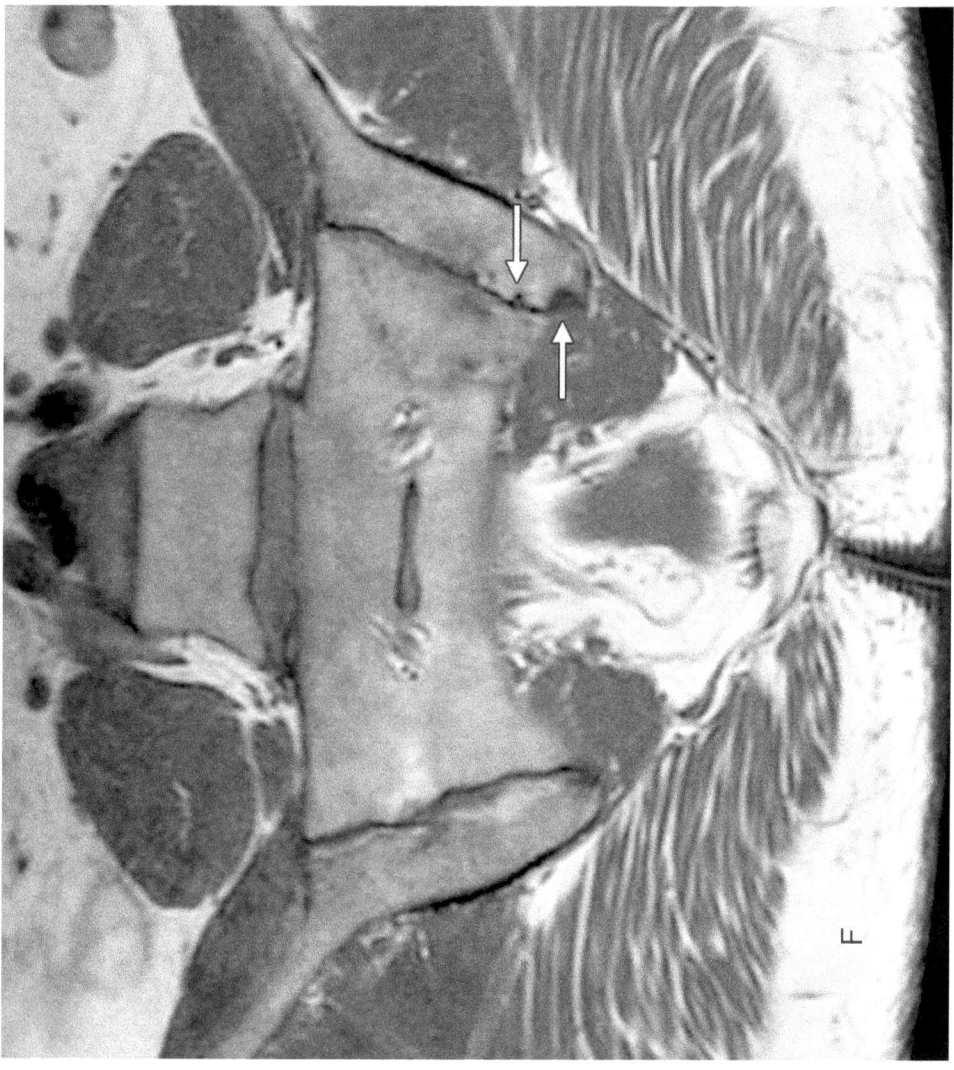

Fig. 43: T1W image (dark intervertebral disc and bright subcutaneous fat [F]) of MRI of SIJ, coronal section showing erosions in the left SIJ (white arrows). T1W sequence is the best to look for erosions.

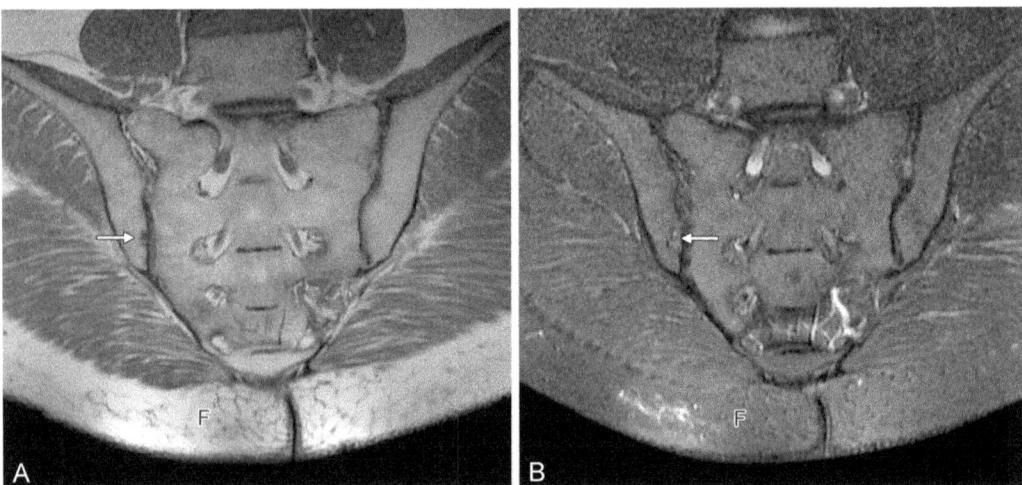

Figs. 44A and B: MRI of SIJ, coronal section showing irregularity of iliac aspect of right SIJ on T1 sequence (white arrow in A) suggestive of erosion. STIR image at the same level shows hyperintense signals within the bony deficit (white arrow in B), which confirms the presence of an erosion. Bright signals are seen within an erosion on STIR sequence due to infiltration of inflammatory cells, in an attempt towards healing.

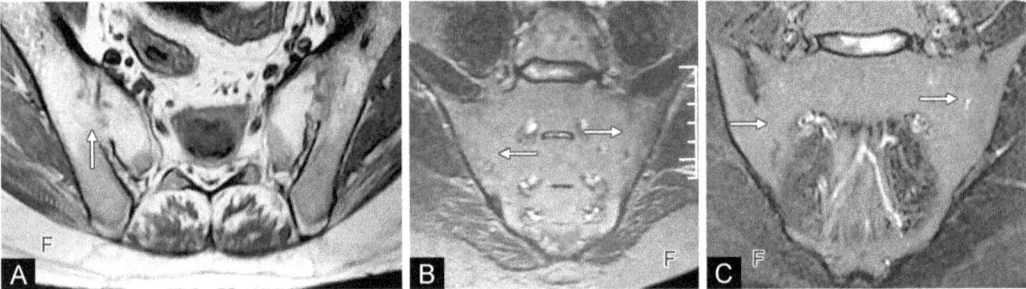

Figs. 45A to C: (A) Axial section of MRI of SIJ showing patchy obliteration of joint space in right SIJ (white arrow), suggestive of ankylosis on T2W MRI (bright subcutaneous fat [F] and CSF); (B) Coronal section of MRI of SIJ showing complete obliteration of both SIJ (white arrows), suggestive of ankylosis on T2W sequence (bright intervertebral disc and subcutaneous fat [F]); (C) Coronal section of MRI of SIJ showing complete obliteration of left SIJ and lower part of right SIJ (white arrows) on STIR (bright intervertebral disc and dark subcutaneous fat [F]).

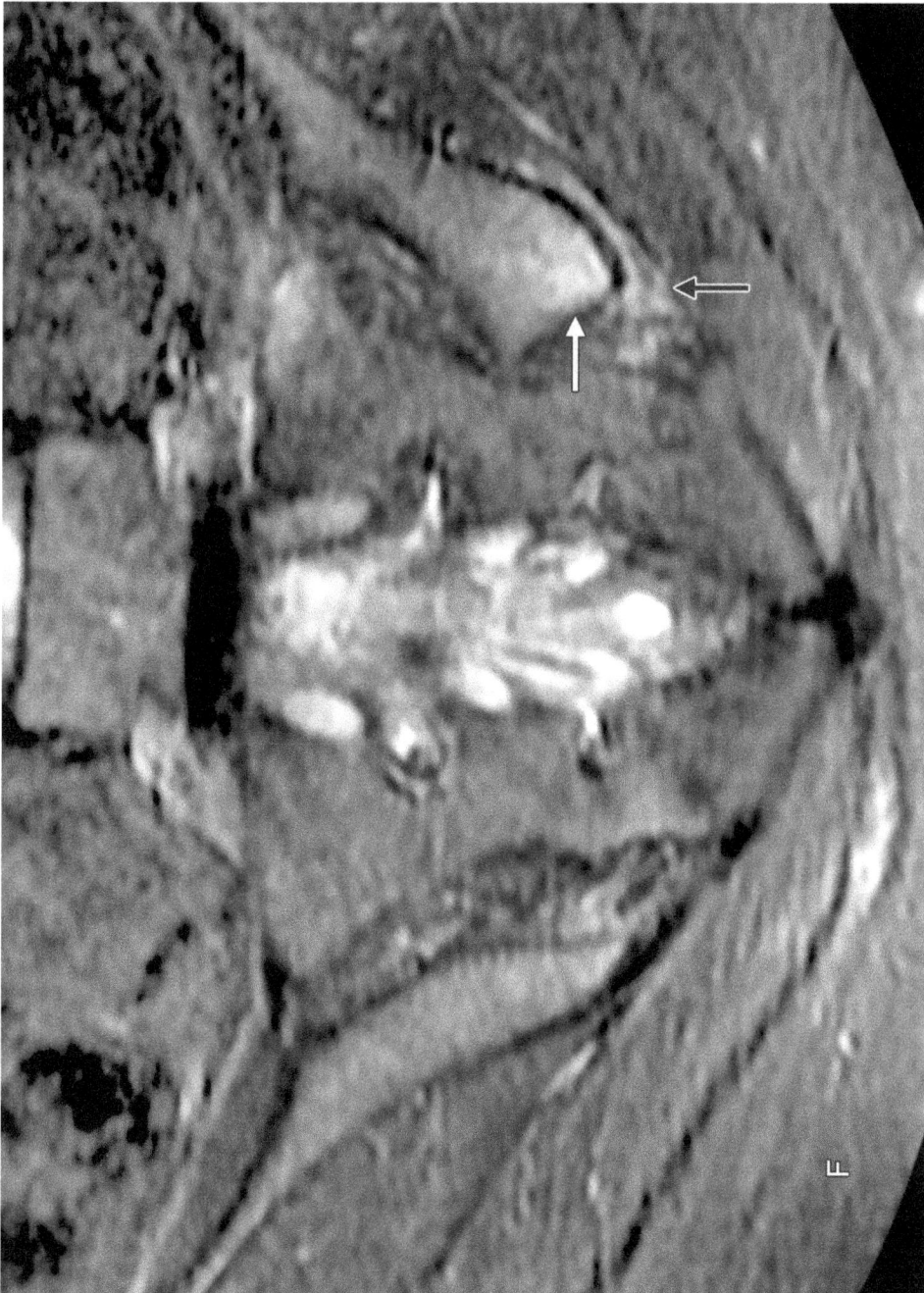

Fig. 46: MRI of SIJ, STIR sequence (dark subcutaneous fat [F]), coronal section showing bright signal intensity in the muscles below the lower margin of left SIJ (black arrow) with bone marrow edema of the underlying ilium (white arrow), suggestive of enthesitis.

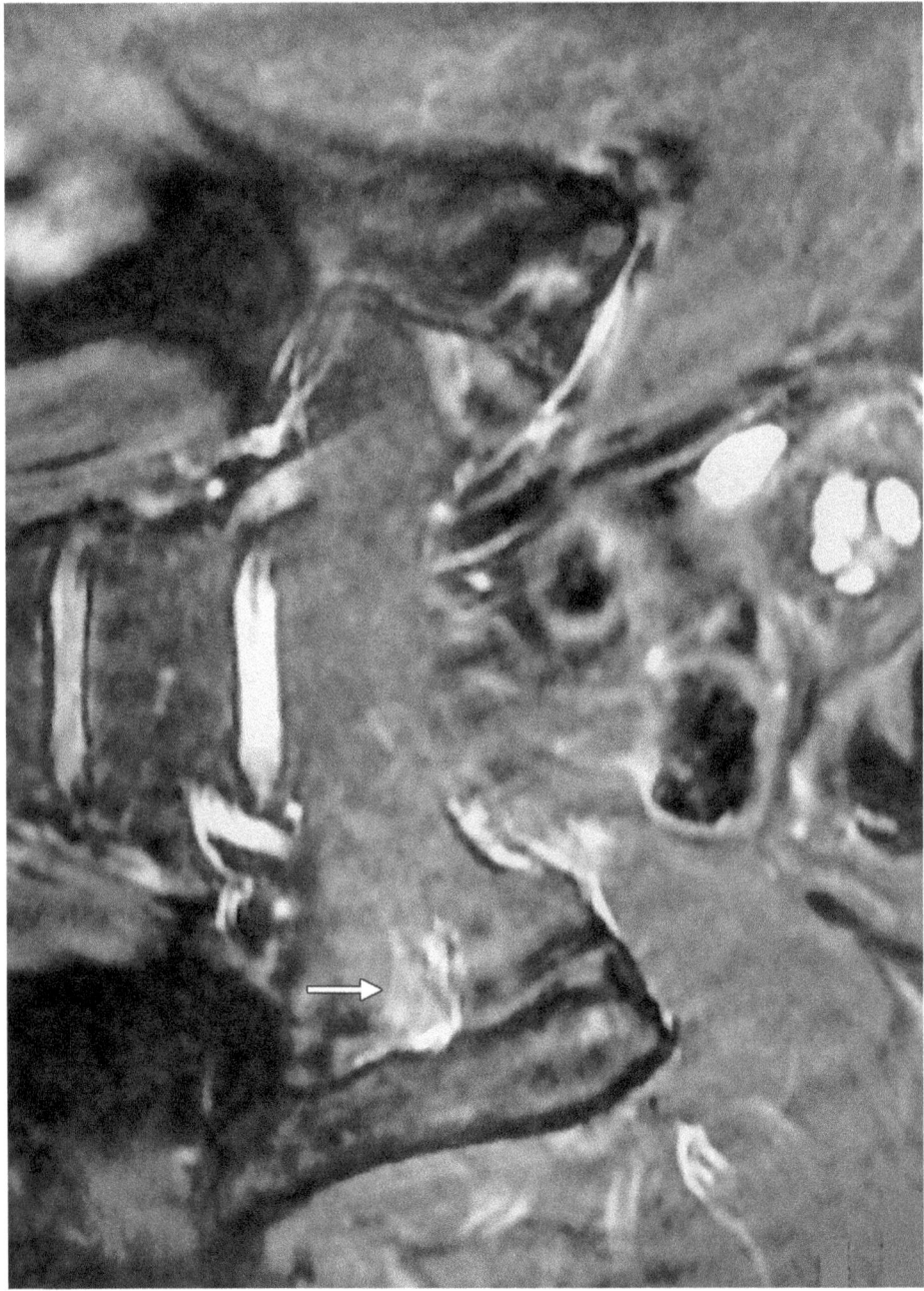

Fig. 47: MRI of SIJ STIR sequence showing bright signal in the upper, ligamentous part of right SIJ (white arrow), suggestive of enthesitis of the ligaments between sacrum and ilium.

MRI OF SPINE

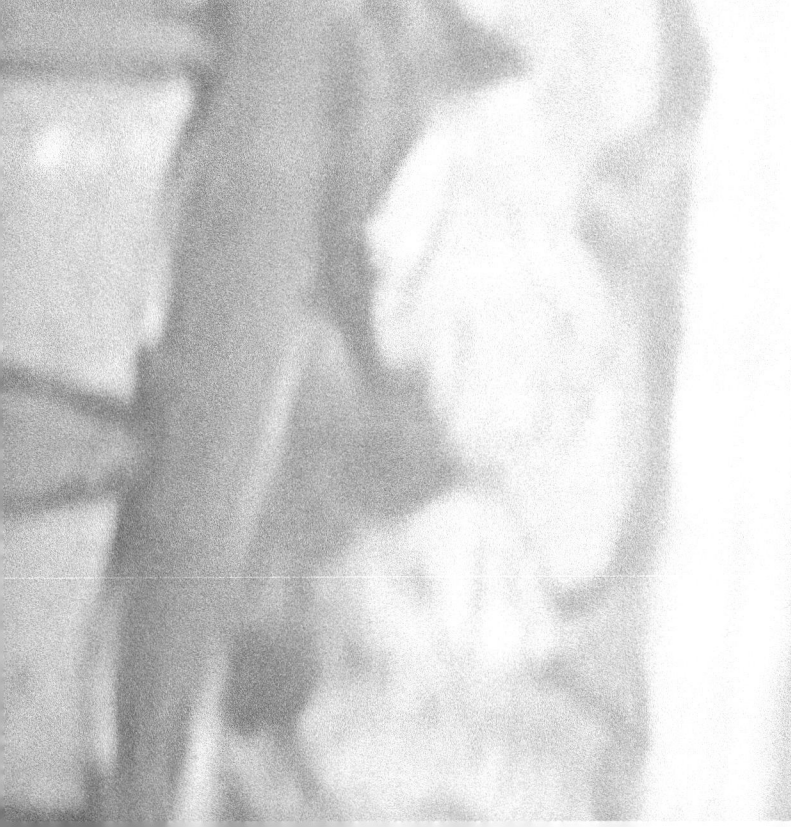

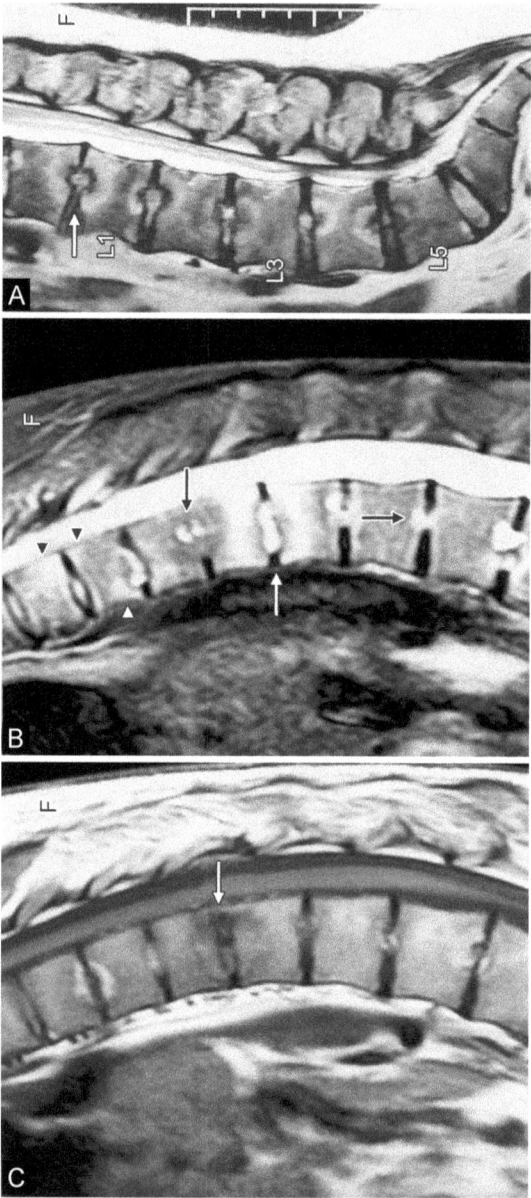

Figs. 48A to C: (A) Sagittal T2W MRI (bright intervertebral discs, CSF and subcutaneous fat [F]) of a young male with non-inflammatory back pain showing Schmorl's nodes, as suggested by the presence of herniation of the nucleus pulposus into the vertebral bodies with surrounding bone marrow edema (white arrow). The bone marrow edema does not involve the end-plate completely, thereby differentiating it from spondylodisciitis (Anderson's lesions); (B) Sagittal STIR MRI (bright intervertebral discs and CSF and dark subcutaneous fat [F]) of a patient with axial-SpA showing irregularity of the vertebral end plate with surrounding bone marrow edema involving the end-plate completely, suggestive of an Anderson's lesion (white arrow). Other lesions as marked by black arrows are Schmorl's nodes; bright signals in the posterior corners (black arrowheads) and anterior corners (white arrowhead) of the vertebral bodies are seen, suggestive of bone marrow edema due to spondylitis (inflammatory corner lesions); (C) Sagittal section of MRI, T1W sequence (dark intervertebral discs and CSF and bright subcutaneous fat) of same patient as in B showing end-plate irregularity and dark signals in the corresponding area as in B, suggestive of bone marrow edema (arrow).

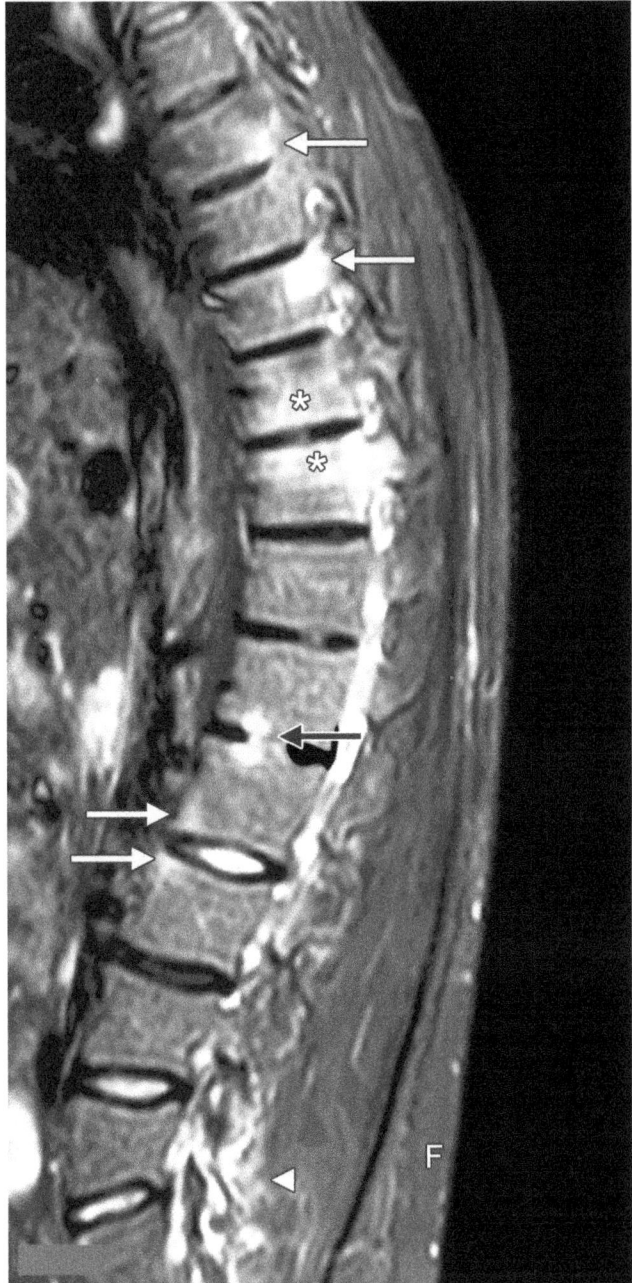

Fig. 49: Sagittal section of MRI of thoracic spine STIR sequence (dark subcutaneous fat [F] and bright intervertebral discs (some of the intervertebral discs are showing dark signals due to co-existing degenerative desiccation of the discs) showing bright signal intensities in the posterior (leftward white arrows) and anterior corners (rightward white arrows) of vertebral bodies, suggestive of bone marrow edema (spondylitis); end-plate bone marrow edema suggestive of spondylodiscitis (asterisks) and bone marrow edema in the posterior elements of vertebrae (white arrowhead), suggestive of facet joint arthropathy. Note is made of a Schmorl's node (black arrow).

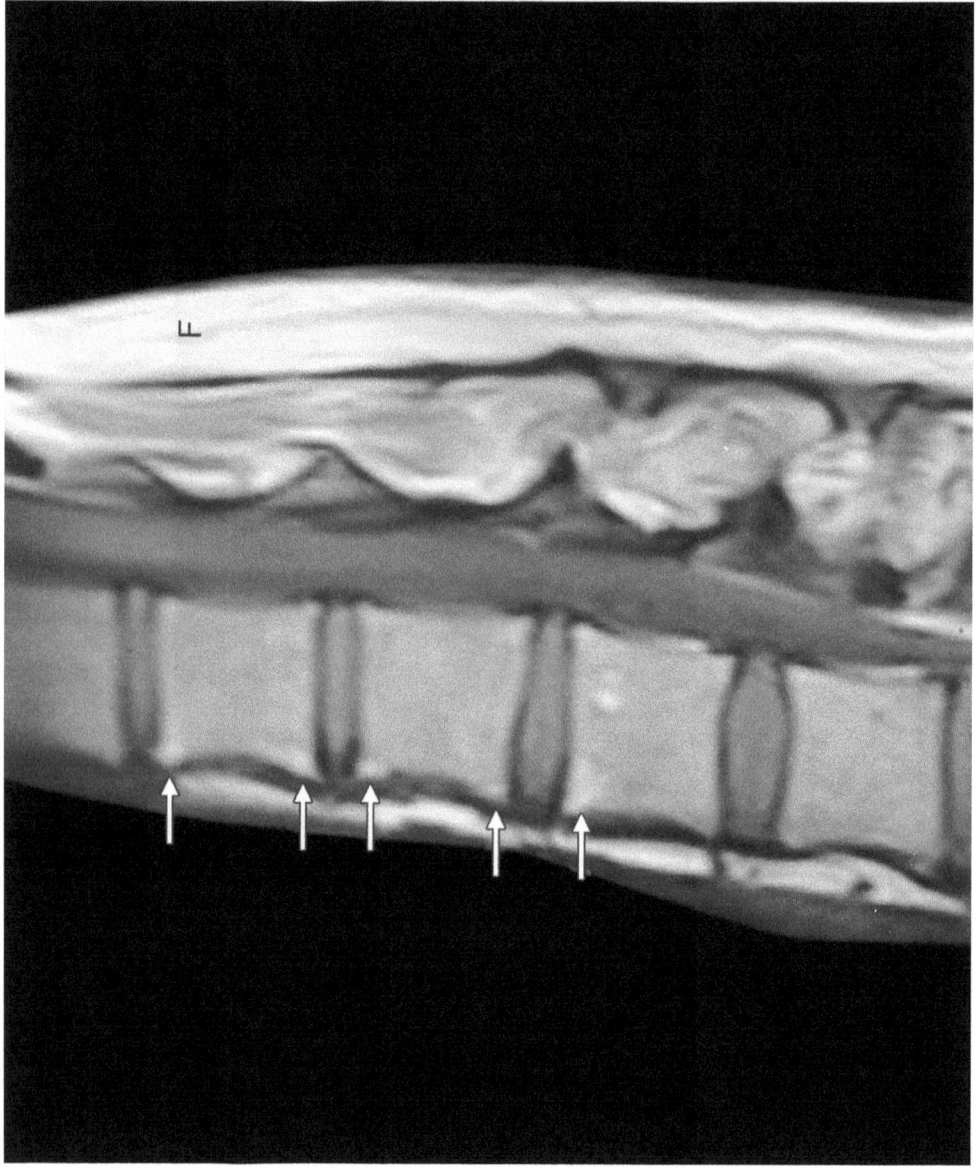

Fig. 50: Sagittal T1W MRI (dark CSF and intervertebral discs and bright subcutaneous fat [F]) showing bright corners in vertebral bodies suggestive of fatty metaplasia (arrows).

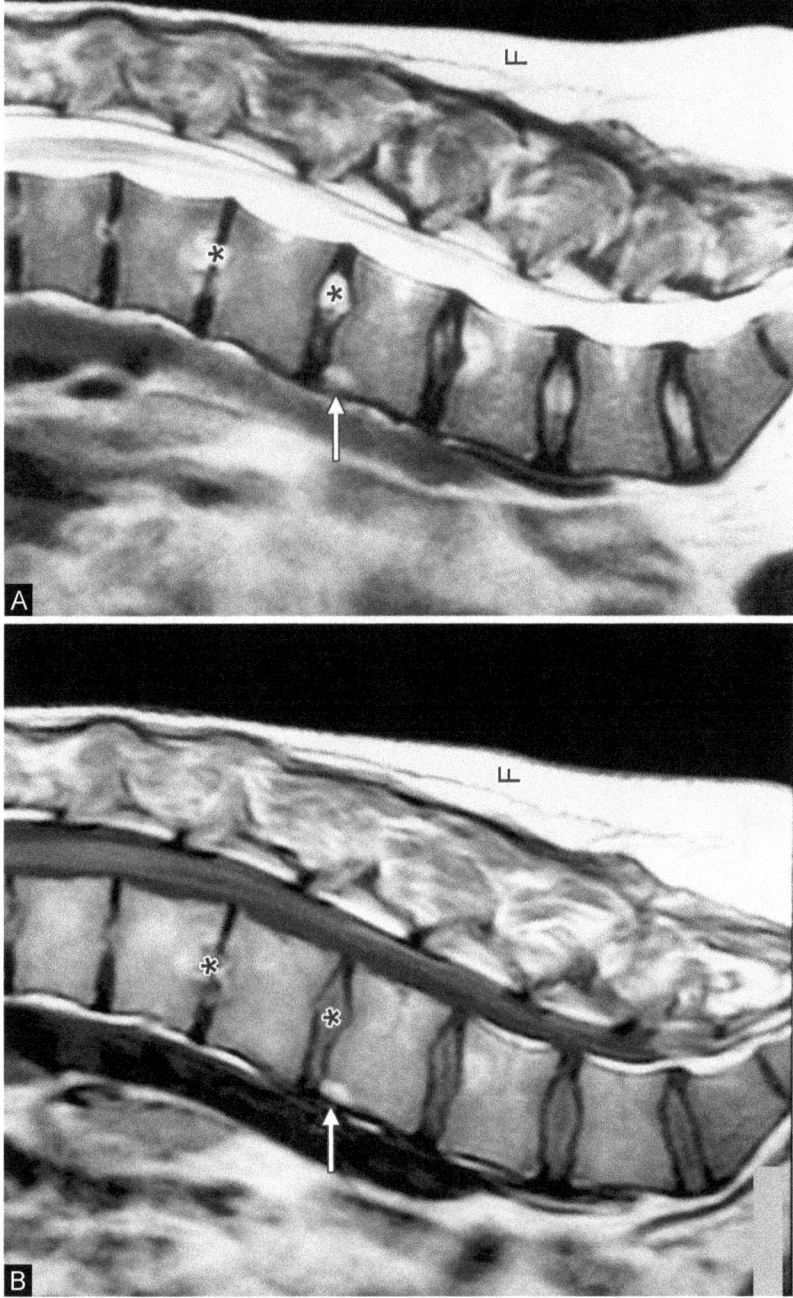

Figs. 51A and B: MRI sagittal section of the lumbar spine. (A) T2W image (bright CSF, intervertebral discs and subcutaneous fat [F]) showing Schmorl's nodes (black asterisks) and bright signal intensity in the upper anterior corner of L3 (white arrow); (B) T1W image of the same patient (dark CSF, intervertebral discs and bright subcutaneous fat [F]) shows the same lesion in L3 which appears bright on T1 also (white arrow). So it is a fatty corner and not bone marrow edema of spondylitis (latter would appear bright on T2 and dark on T1). Schmorl's nodes are marked by asterisks.

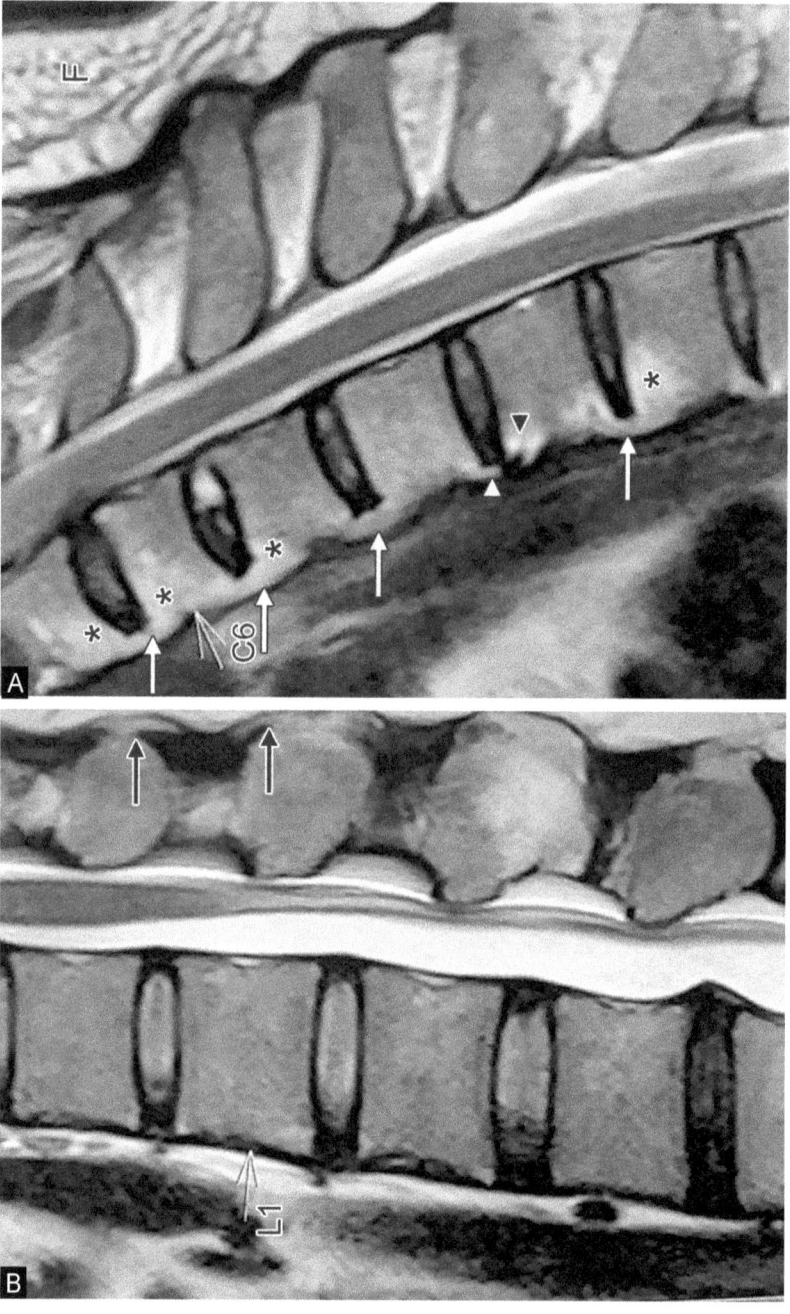

Figs. 52A and B: Sagittal section of MRI of spine, T2W sequences (bright intervertebral discs, CSF and subcutaneous fat [F]). (A) Bridging (white arrows) and non-bridging (white arrowheads) syndesmophytes. Note that sydesmophytes are developing at the sites of fatty metaplasia (asterisks). An erosion is seen at the upper anterior corner of T2 vertebral body (black arrowhead); (B) Patchy calcification of supraspinous ligament (black arrows) is observed.

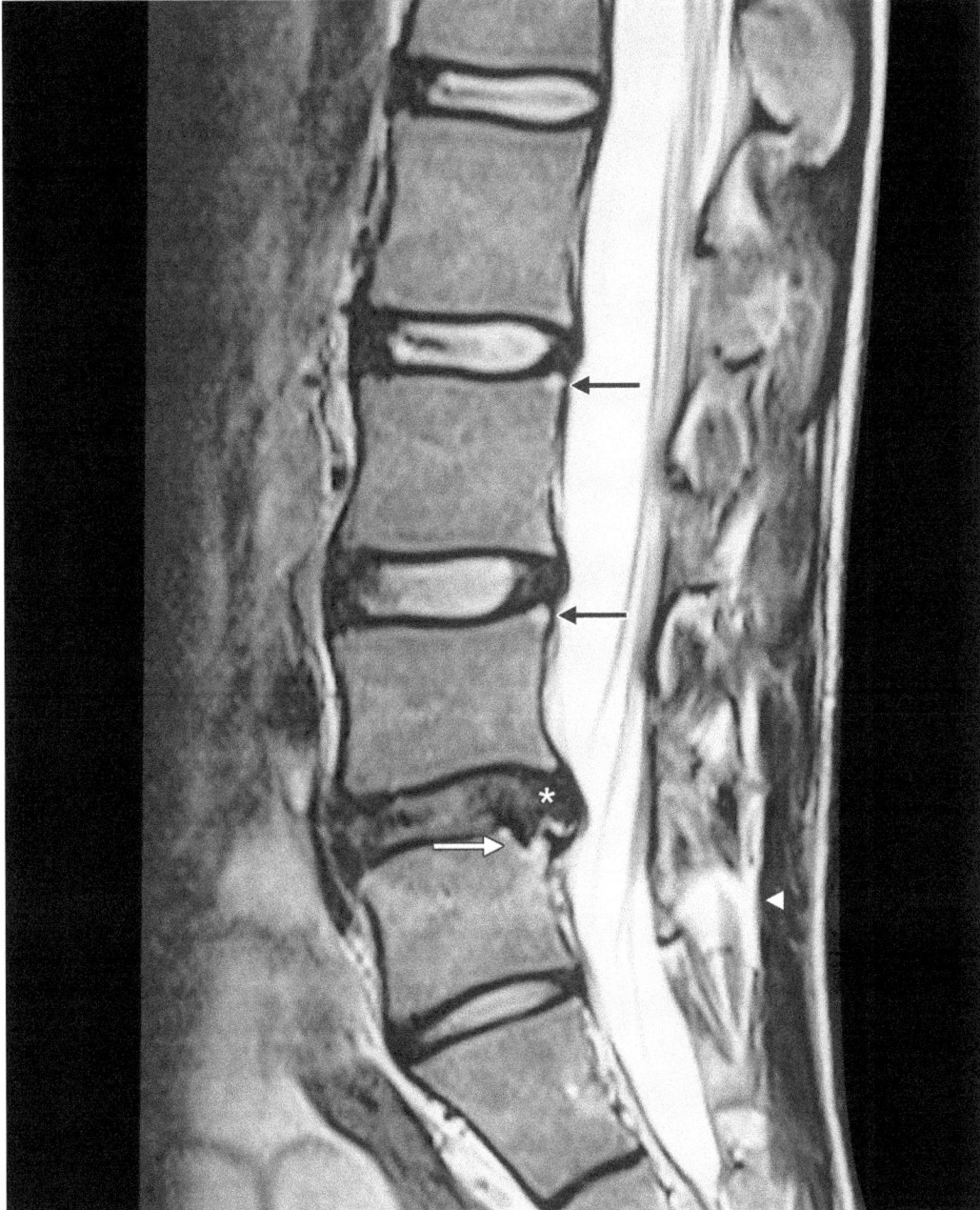

Fig. 53: MRI of lumbar spine, sagittal section, T2 sequence showing erosion in the posterior upper corner of L5 (white arrow); desiccated and prolapsed intervertebral disc between L4 and L5 (asterisk); small areas of fatty metaplasia at posterior corners of L3 and L4 (black arrows); bright signals in the posterior elements of the vertebrae, suggestive of facet joint arthritis (white arrowhead).

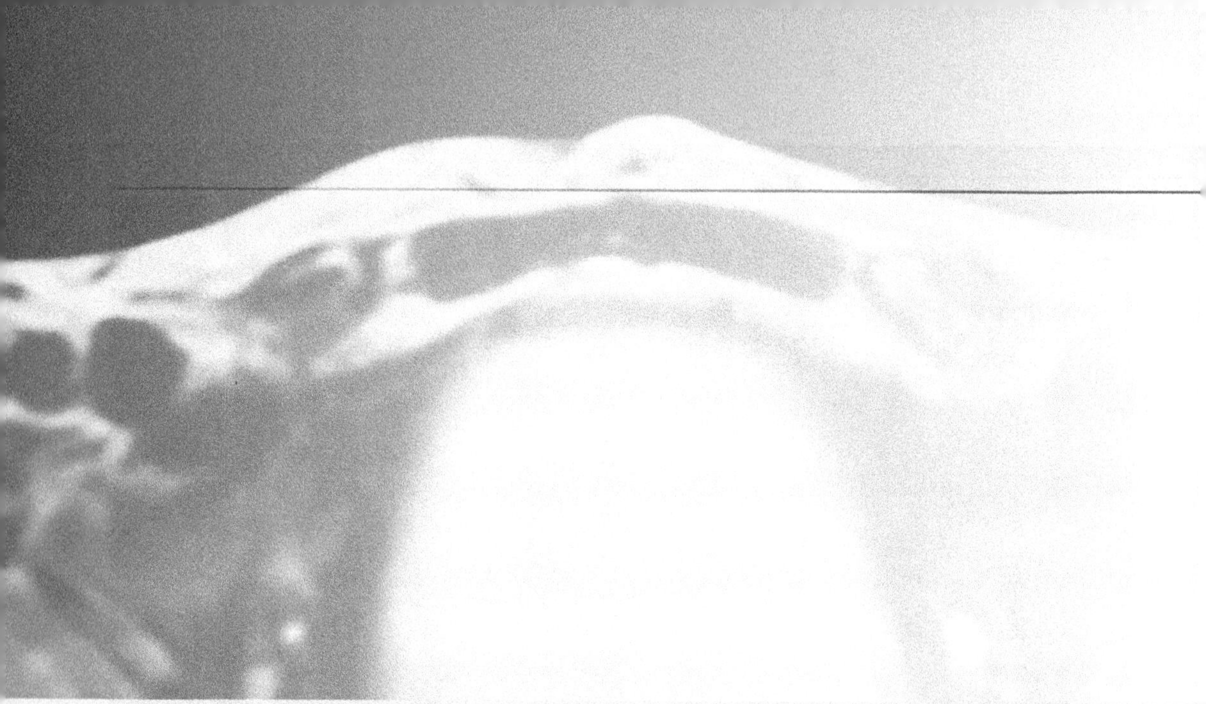

INFECTIONS MIMICKING SpA

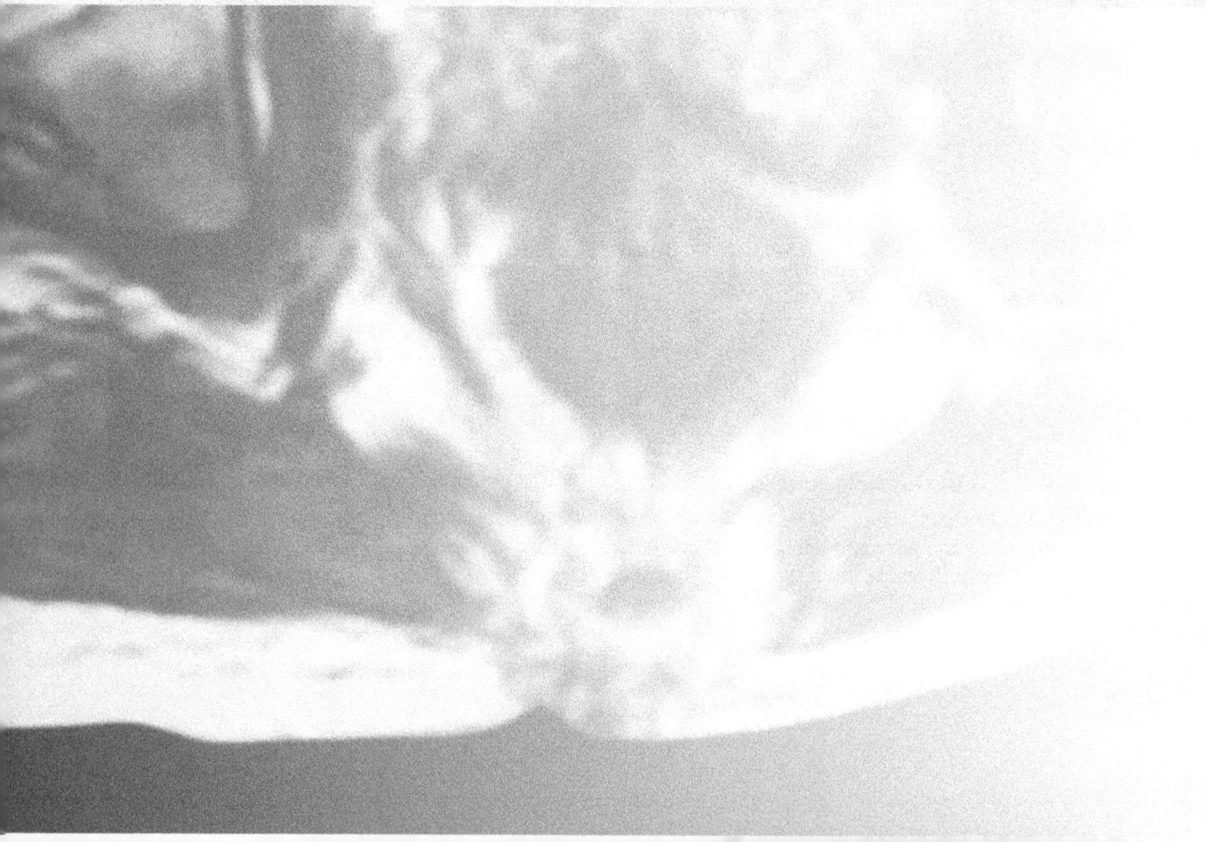

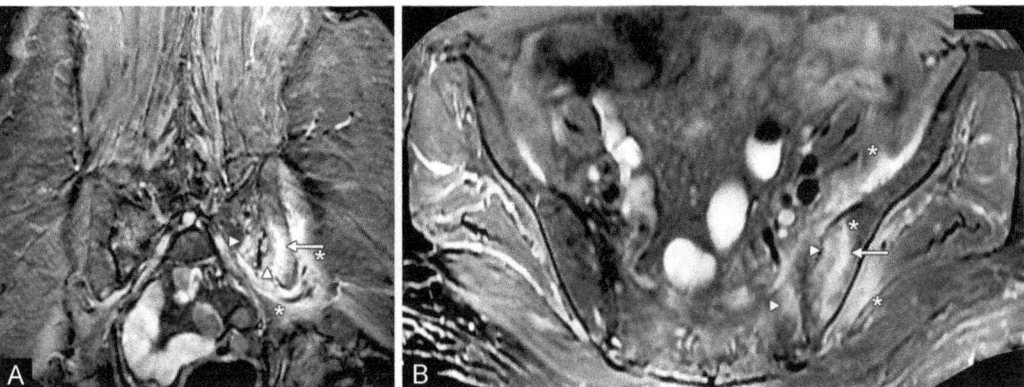

Figs. 54A and B: MRI of pelvis, STIR sequences showing bone marrow edema on the sacral and iliac aspects of left SIJ, suggestive of sacroiliitis (white arrowheads). Note that the edema extends beyond the anatomic boundaries of SIJ (white asterisks). In addition, the area of maximum hyperintensity is away from the subarticular area of the ilium (white arrows). These features point against SpA as the etiology of sacroiliitis. Biopsy from left SIJ showed granulomatous inflammation with positive ZN stain for AFB, suggestive of tubercular sacroiliitis. (A) Coronal; (B) Axial.

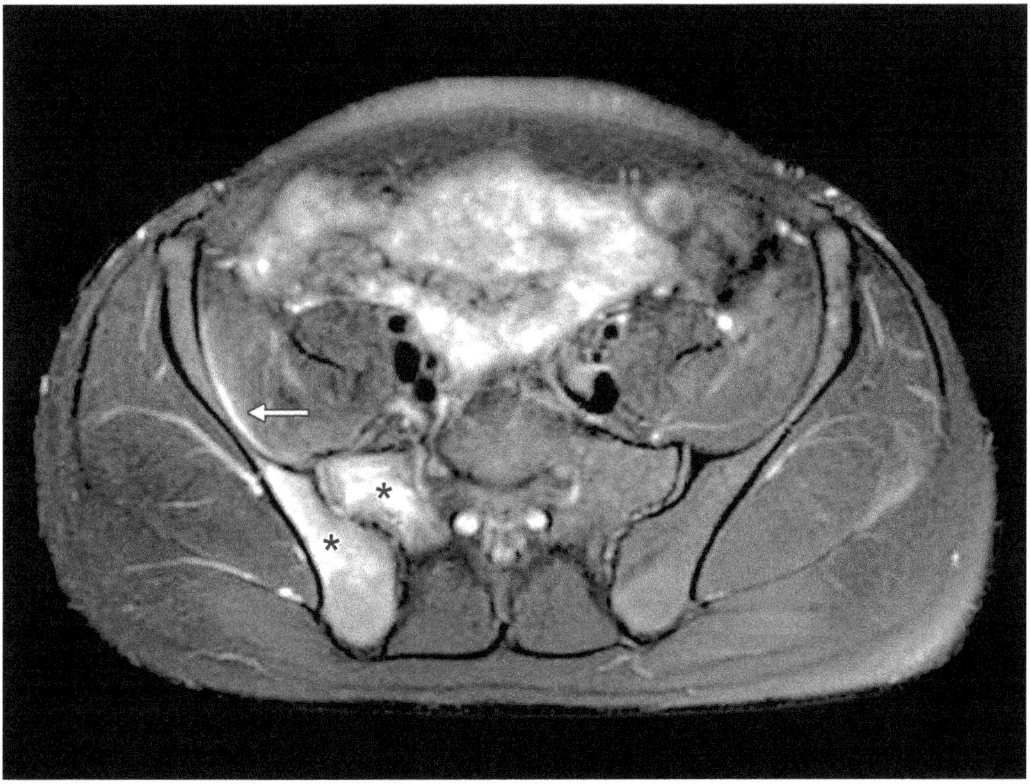

Fig. 55: MRI of SIJ, STIR sequence, axial section showing bright signals in sacral and iliac aspects of right SIJ (asterisks), suggestive of bone marrow edema. Edema extends beyond the anatomical boundaries of right SIJ into right iliacus muscle (arrow), which suggests infection.[16] Biopsy from right SIJ showed necrosis with positive ZN staining for AFB, suggestive of tubercular sacroiliitis.

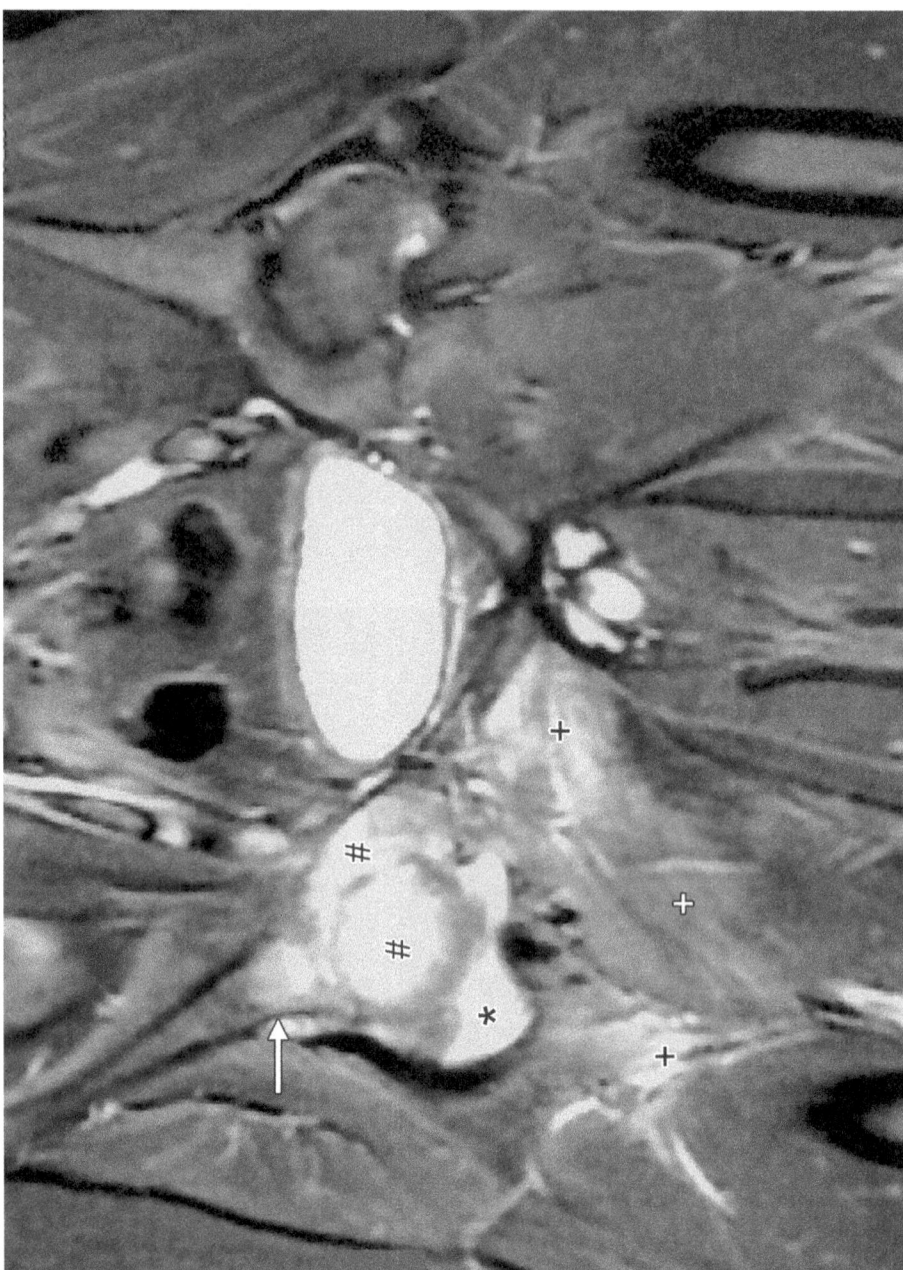

Fig. 56: STIR sequence of MRI of a known case of AS with right hip pain showing effusion in the right hip joint (asterisk), intense bone marrow edema in head of femur and acetabulum on the right side (hash). Bone marrow edema extends beyond the anatomic boundaries of the right hip joint involving the lowest part of right ilium (white arrow) and the muscles of the upper part of the thigh are also edematous (bright signal intensity in muscles) (plus marks). These features are suggestive of an infection. Synovial biopsy showed granulomatous inflammation with positive PCR for *Mycobacterium tuberculosis*.

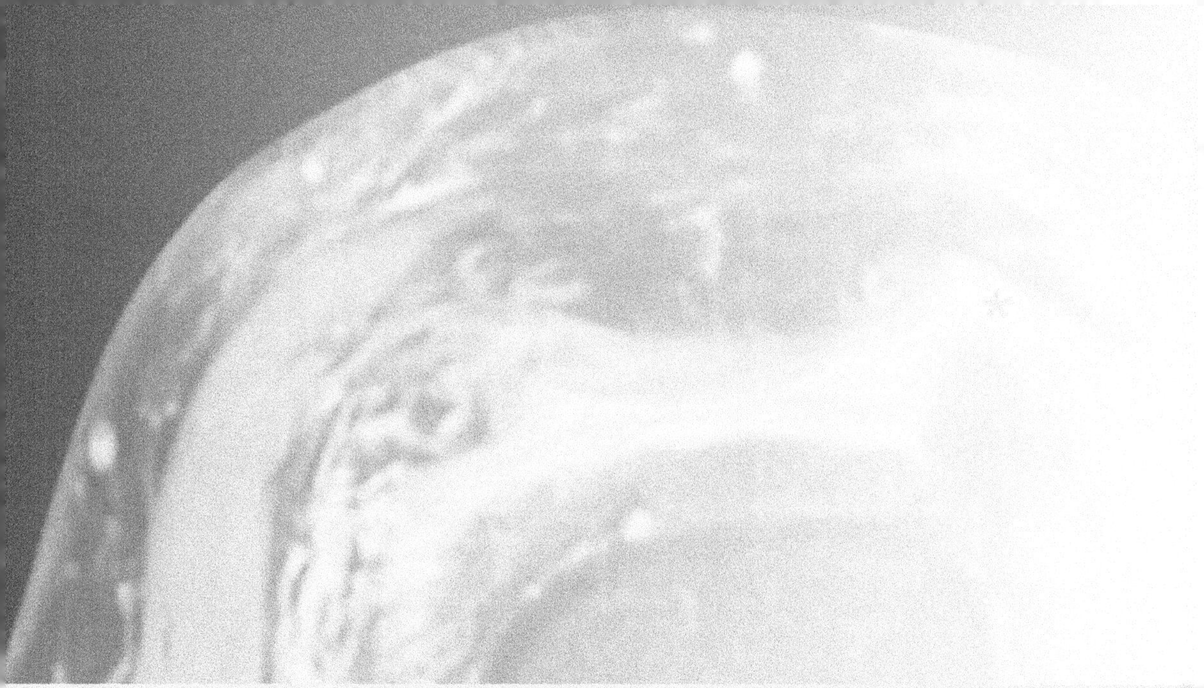

MRI OF PERIPHERAL JOINTS

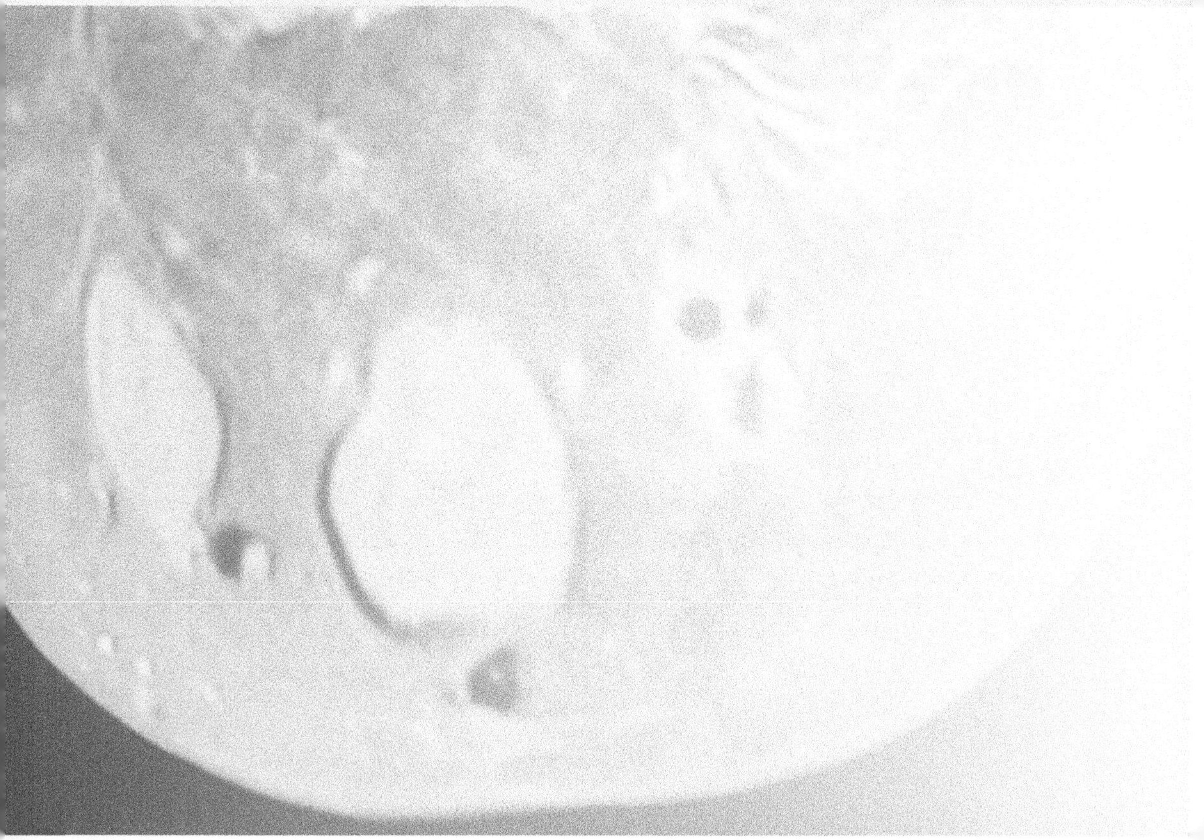

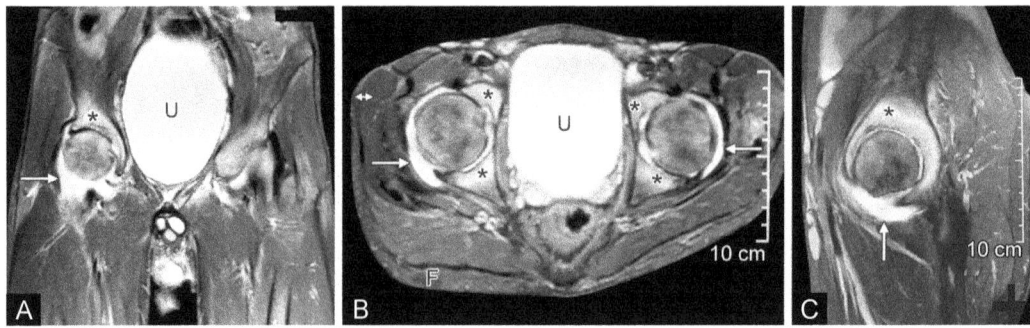

Figs. 57A to C: MRI of the pelvis, STIR sequences (bright urine [U] and dark subcutaneous fat [F]) of a patient with peripheral SpA (A: coronal section, B: axial section, C: sagittal section) showing bright (fluid) signal intensity around the hip joint suggestive of joint effusion (white arrows in A, B and C); bright signal intensity in the acetabulum above the head of the femur in A and C and medial to head of femur on both sides in B (black asterisks), suggestive of acetabular bone marrow edema.

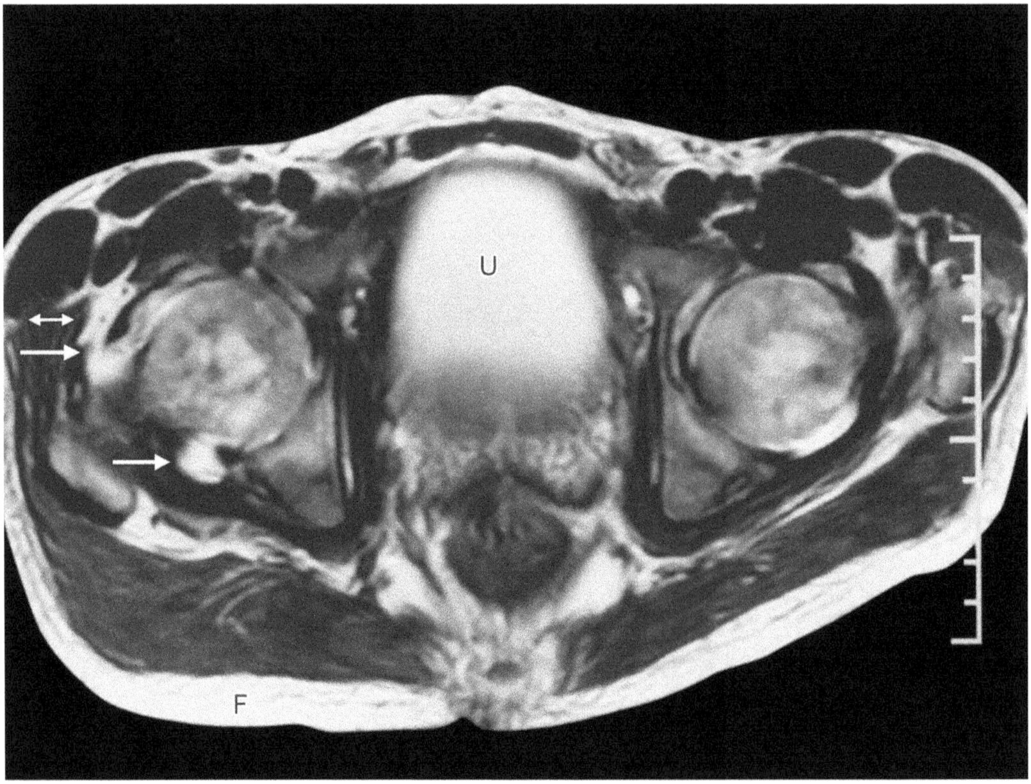

Fig. 58: Axial section of T2W MRI (urine [U] and subcutaneous fat [F] are bright) showing bright signal intensity of the reflection of the capsule of the right hip joint over the neck of femur (white arrows), suggestive of capsulitis.

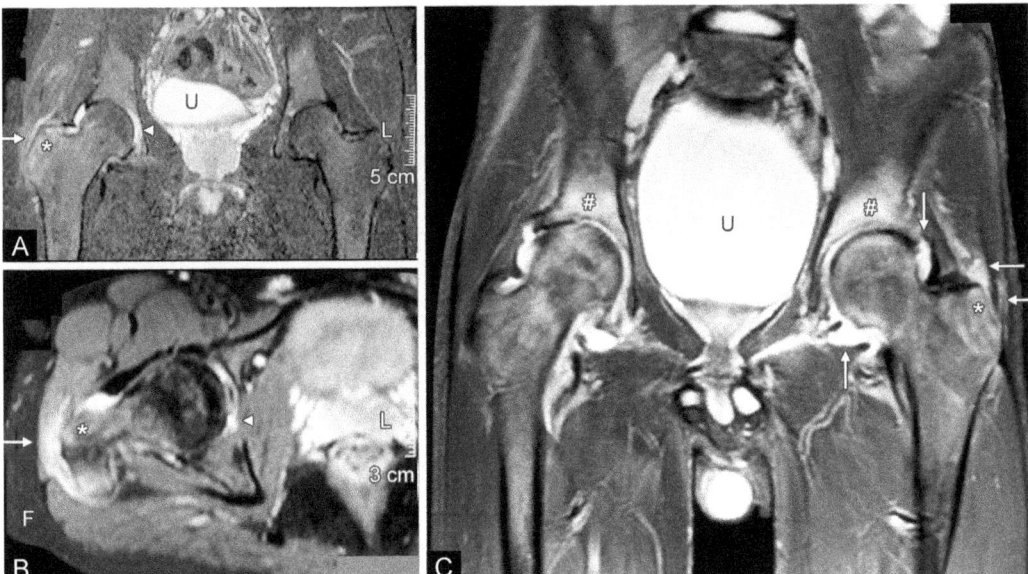

Figs. 59A to C: (A and B) MRI of the pelvis STIR sequences (dark subcutaneous fat [F] and bright urine [U]) of the same patient showing bright signal intensity in the right gluteal tendons near their attachment at the right greater trochanter (horizontal white arrows) with bone marrow edema in the subjacent greater trochanter (white asterisks) suggestive of enthesitis. A note is made of mild right hip joint effusion (white arrowheads) (A: coronal, B: axial); (C) Coronal section of the MRI of pelvis (STIR) of another patient showing bright signal intensity in the tendons near their attachment at the left greater trochanter (horizontal white arrows) with bone marrow edema of the left greater trochanter (white asterisk) suggestive of enthesitis; bright signal intensity of the reflection of the joint capsule of left hip joint suggestive of capsulitis (vertical white arrows); hyperintense signal intensity in the supra-acetabular regions suggestive of bone marrow edema (hash).

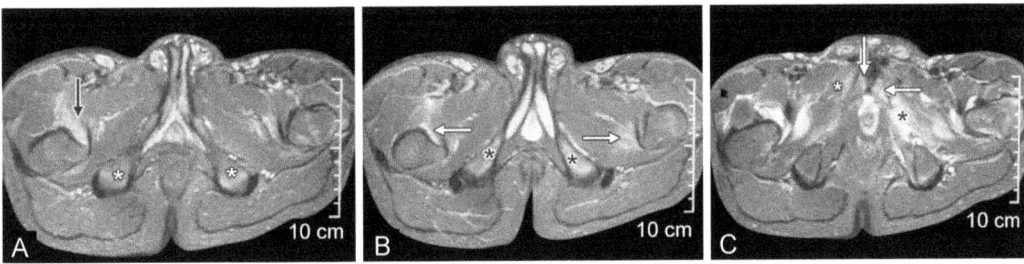

Figs. 60A to C: Coronal sections of STIR sequences of MRI through lower pelvis showing: (A) Bone marrow edema in ischial tuberosities (white asterisks) with edema of the myotendinous junctions of muscles attaching at the right lesser trochanter suggestive of enthesitis (black arrow); (B) Bone marrow edema in both inferior pubic rami (black asterisks) and edema of the myotendinous junctions of muscles attaching at the lesser trochanter on both sides suggestive of enthesitis (white arrows); (C) Edema of the muscles around the left inferior pubic ramus (black asterisk) and right pubic symphysis (white asterisk) and bone marrow edema in pubic symphysis (white arrows) suggestive of enthesitis.

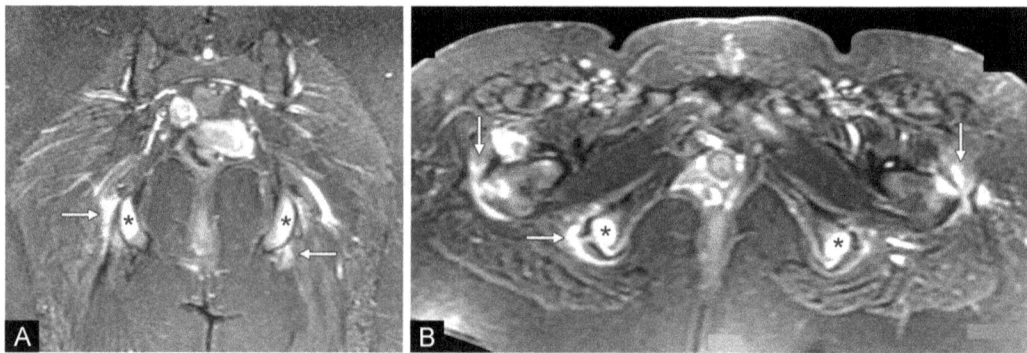

Figs. 61A and B: MRI of pelvis, STIR sequence showing bright signal intensity in both ischial tuberosities (black asterisks) and the muscles around (horizontal white arrows), suggestive of enthesitis. Note is also made of enthesitis in both greater trochanters (vertical white arrows in B). (A) Coronal section, (B) Axial section.

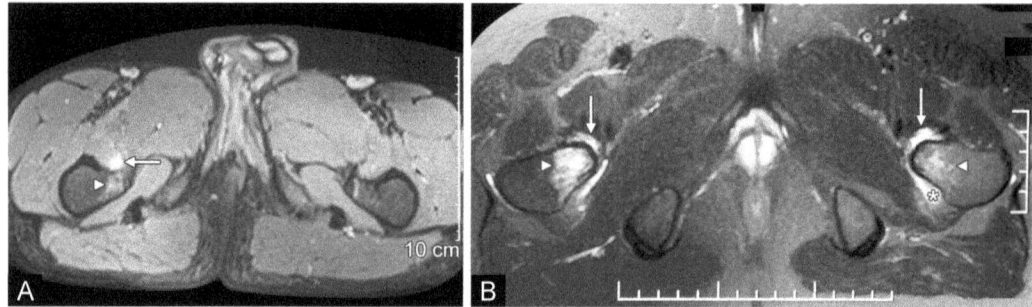

Figs. 62A and B: (A) Axial section of STIR sequence of MRI of pelvis showing bright signals in the muscles near the attachment to the lesser trochanter on right side (white arrow) with bone marrow edema in the lesser trochanter (white arrowhead), suggestive of enthesitis; (B) Similar changes on both sides in another patient with mild effusion on left side (white asterisk).

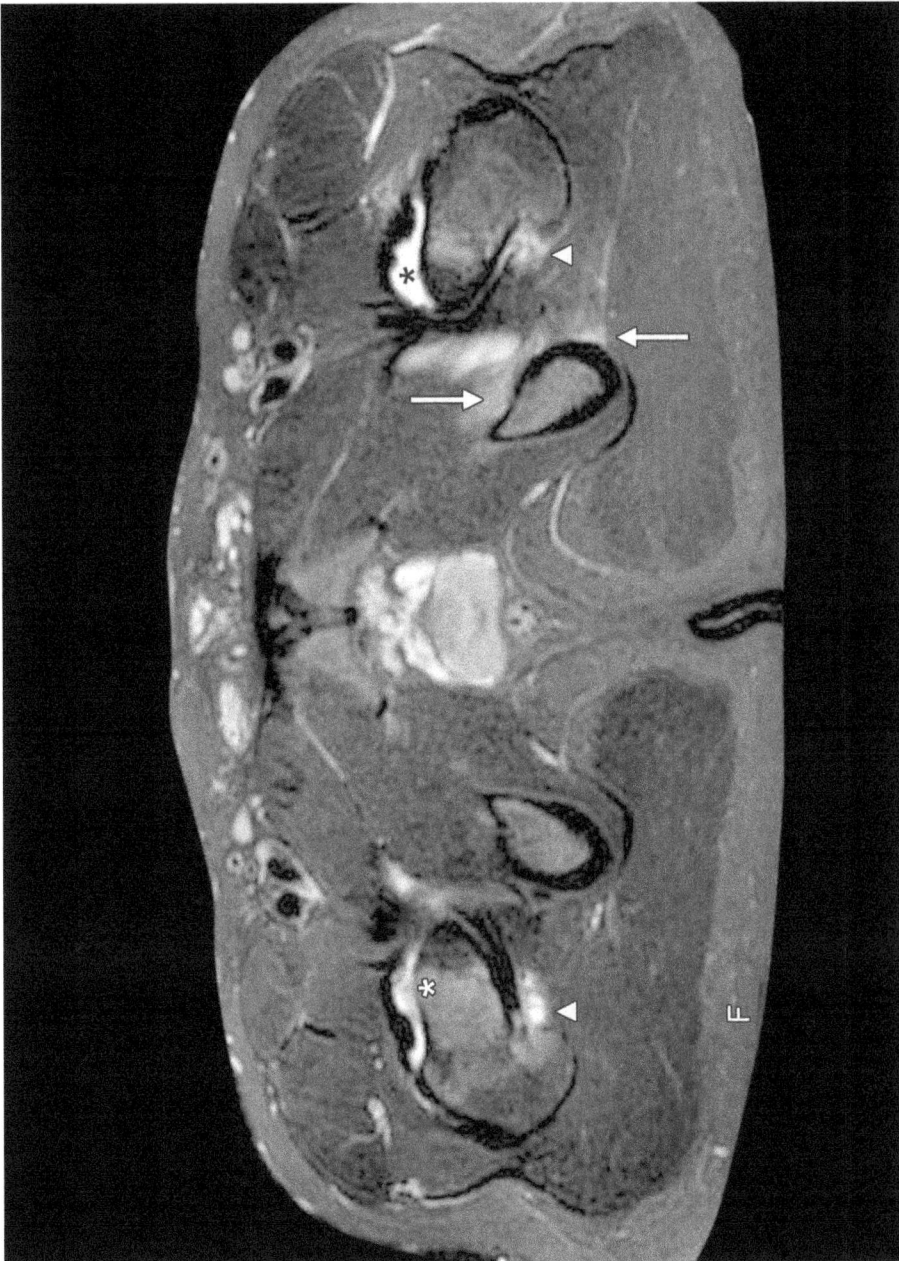

Fig. 63: MRI of pelvis, axial section, STIR sequence (dark subcutaneous fat [F]) showing bright signals in the tendons of muscles attaching to the left ischial tuberosity (white arrows) and both greater trochanters (white arrowheads) suggestive of enthesitis. Note is also made of mild subtrochantric effusion on both sides (asterisks).

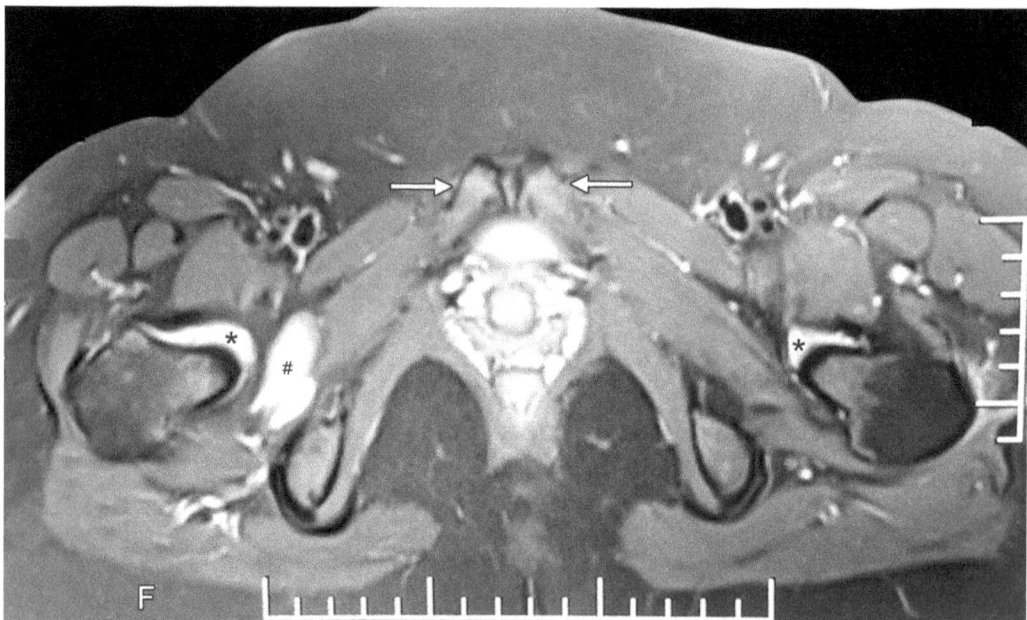

Fig. 64: Axial section of MRI of the pelvis, STIR sequence (dark subcutaneous fat [F]) showing bone marrow edema in both pubic symphyses (white arrows) suggestive of enthesitis with iliopsoas bursitis on the right side (hash). Note is made of mild bilateral hip joint effusion (asterisks).

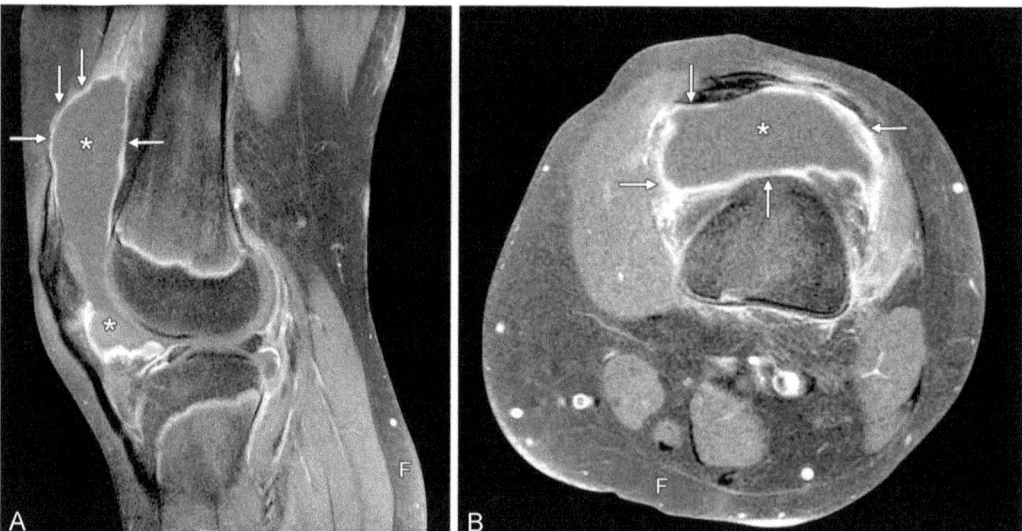

Figs. 65A and B: (A) Sagittal section of contrast-enhanced, fat-suppressed T1W MRI (synovial effusion is dark [white asterisk] and subcutaneous fat is also dark [F]) of the knee joint of a 9-year old girl with enthesitis related arthritis variant of JIA showing a large joint effusion extending into the suprapatellar bursa (white asterisk) with contrast enhancement of the synovial membrane surrounding the effusion, suggestive of synovitis (white arrows); (B) Contrast-enhanced, fat-suppressed T1W sequence of the same patient in axial section showing joint effusion (white asterisk) and synovitis (white arrows).

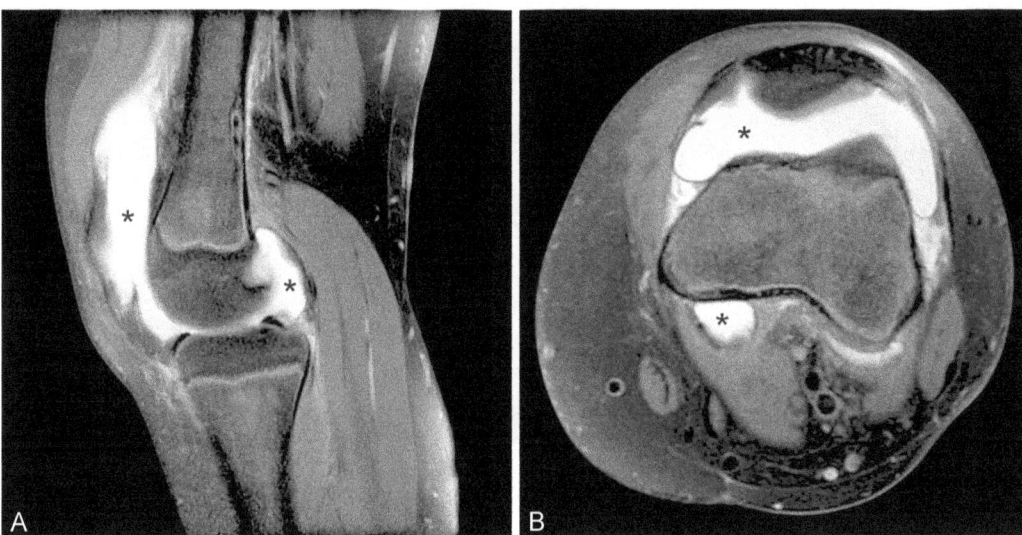

Figs. 66A and B: Sagittal section (A) and coronal section (B) of MRI of knee, STIR sequence of the same patient as in Figure 65, showing knee joint effusion extending into the suprapatellar bursa (black asterisks).

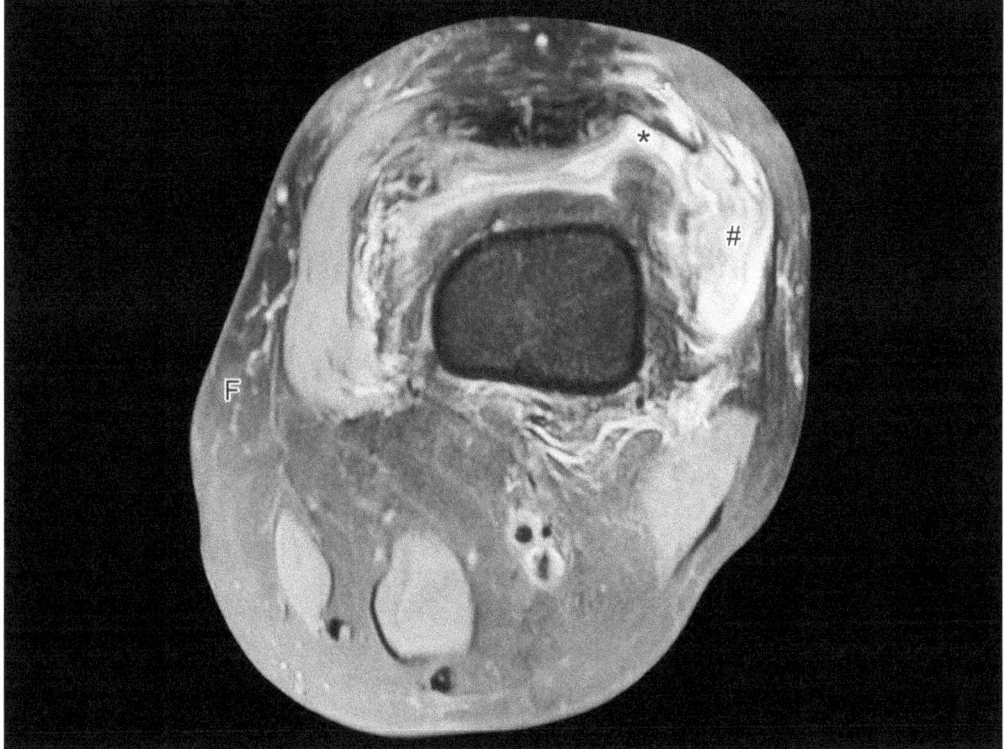

Fig. 67: MRI of knee, axial section, STIR sequence (joint effusion is bright (black asterisk) and subcutaneous fat is dark [F]) of a patient with axial and peripheral SpA showing joint effusion (black asterisk) and synovitis and synovial hypertrophy (hash).

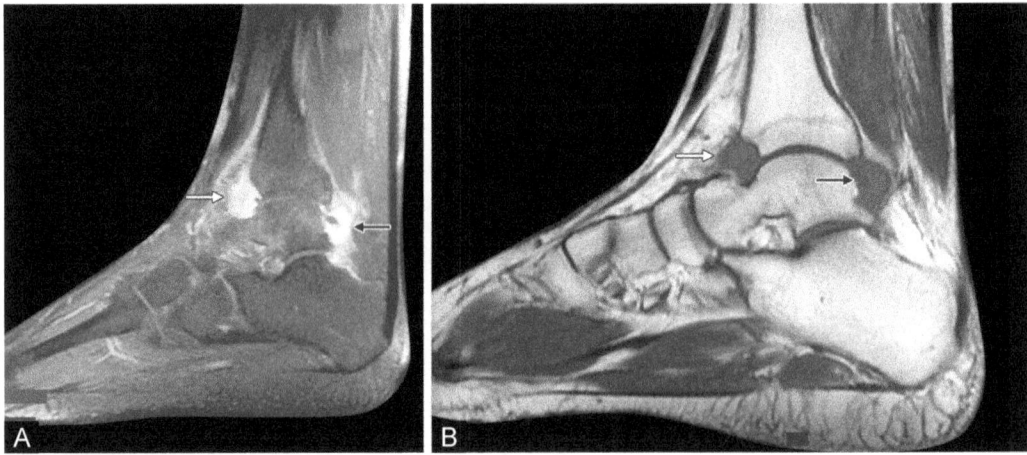

Figs. 68A and B: MRI of ankle, sagittal sections showing effusion of the tibiotalar joint. (A) Bright signal intensity in the anterior (white arrow) and posterior (black arrow) recesses of the tibiotalar joint on STIR sequence, suggestive of joint effusion; (B) T1W sequence showing dark signal intensity in the anterior (white arrow) and posterior (black arrow) recesses of the tibiotalar joint, suggestive of joint effusion.

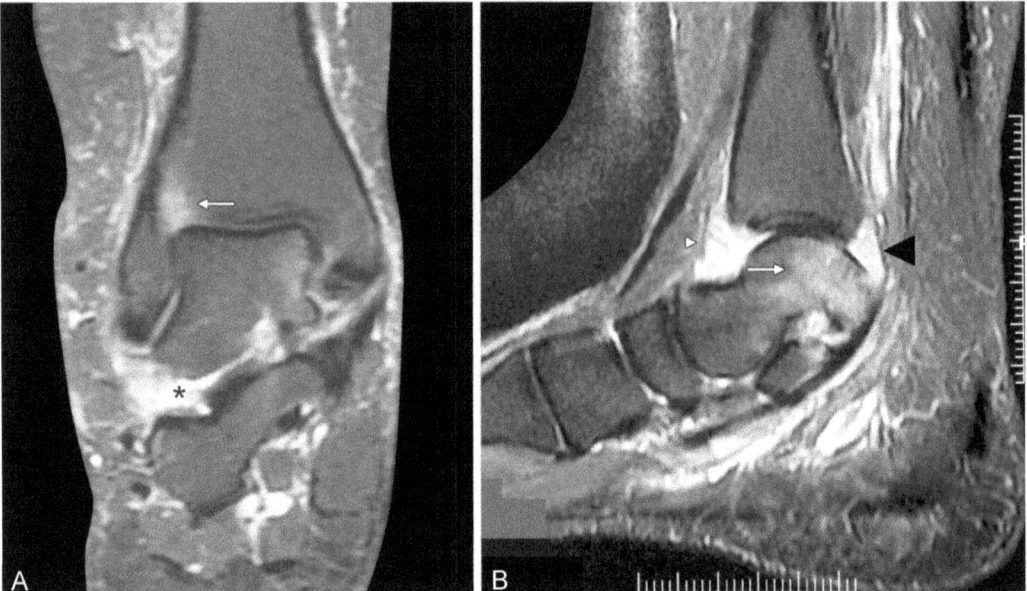

Figs. 69A and B: MRI of ankle, STIR sequences of a young male with peripheral SpA showing bright signal in the lower end of tibia (white arrow in A), bright signal in the posterior part of talus (white arrow in B), suggestive of bone marrow edema. Note is also made of effusion in the subtalar joint in A (black asterisk) and effusion in anterior (white arrowhead) and posterior (black arrowhead) recesses of the tibiotalar joint in B. (A) Coronal section; (B) Sagittal section.

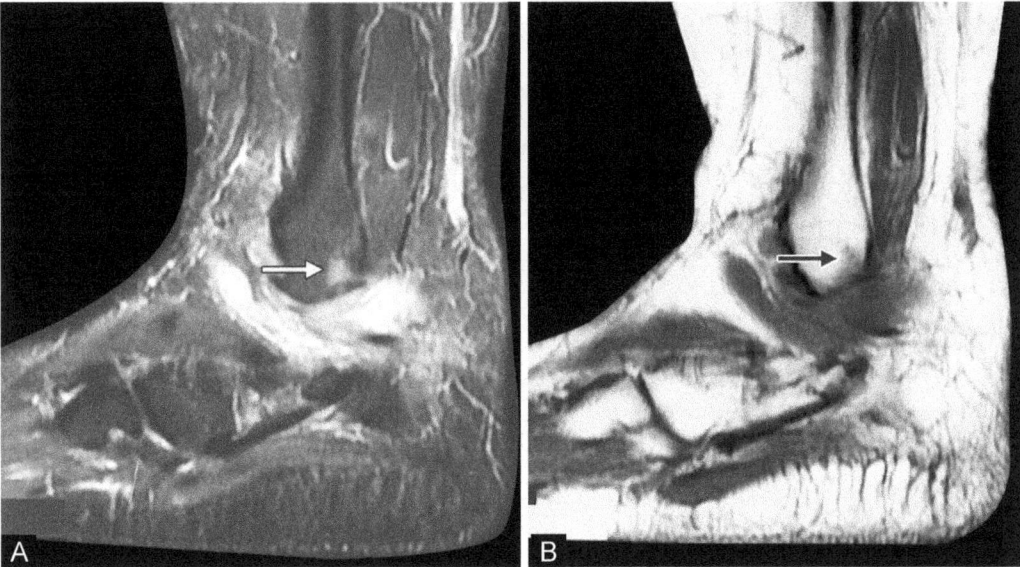

Figs. 70A and B: Sagittal sections of MRI of ankle showing a focal bright signal intensity in the lower part of fibula on STIR sequence (white arrow in A) and dark signal in the corresponding area on T1 (black arrow in B), suggestive of erosion.

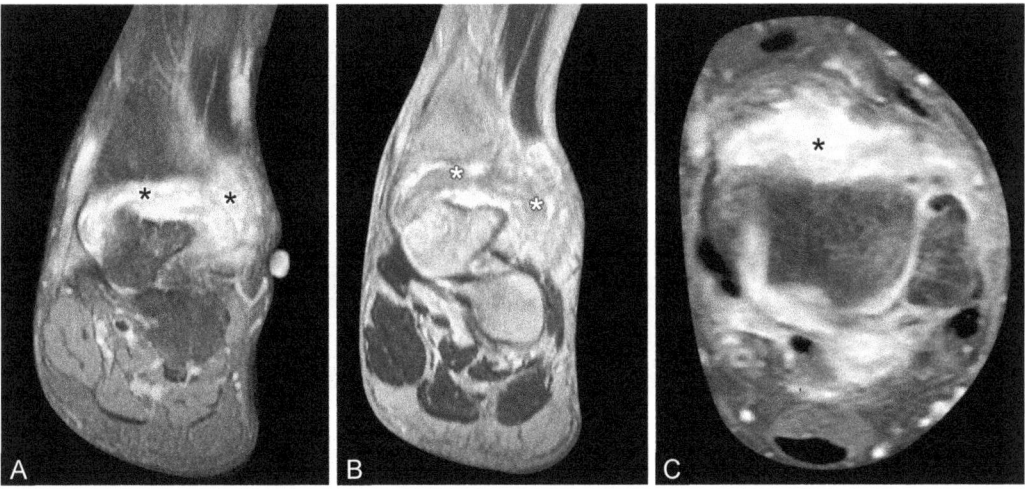

Figs. 71A to C: MRI of ankle of a patient with chronic peripheral SpA showing synovial hypertrophy. (A) Coronal section, STIR sequence showing heterogeneous signal intensity in the tibiotalar joint (black asterisks) with marked increase in the thickness of the synovium, suggestive of synovial hypertrophy; (B) T2W sequence of the corresponding area as in A showing synovial hypertrophy (white asterisks); (C) Axial section, STIR sequence showing heterogeneous signal intensity in the anterior aspect of the tibiotalar joint (black asterisk), suggestive of synovial hypertrophy.

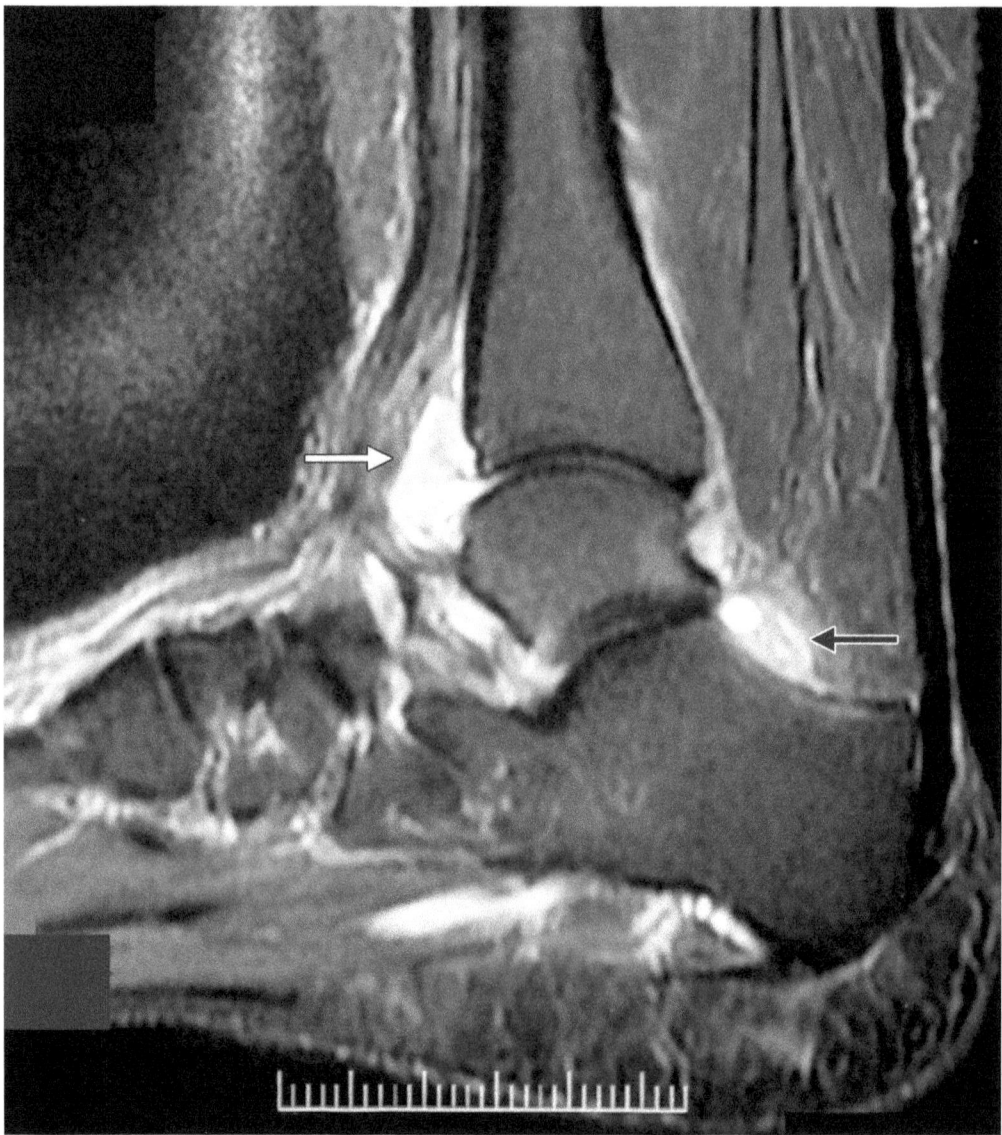

Fig. 72: Sagittal section of MRI of ankle, STIR sequence showing heterogeneous signal intensity in the anterior (white arrow) and posterior (black arrow) recesses of the tibiotalar joint, suggestive of effusion with synovial hypertrophy.

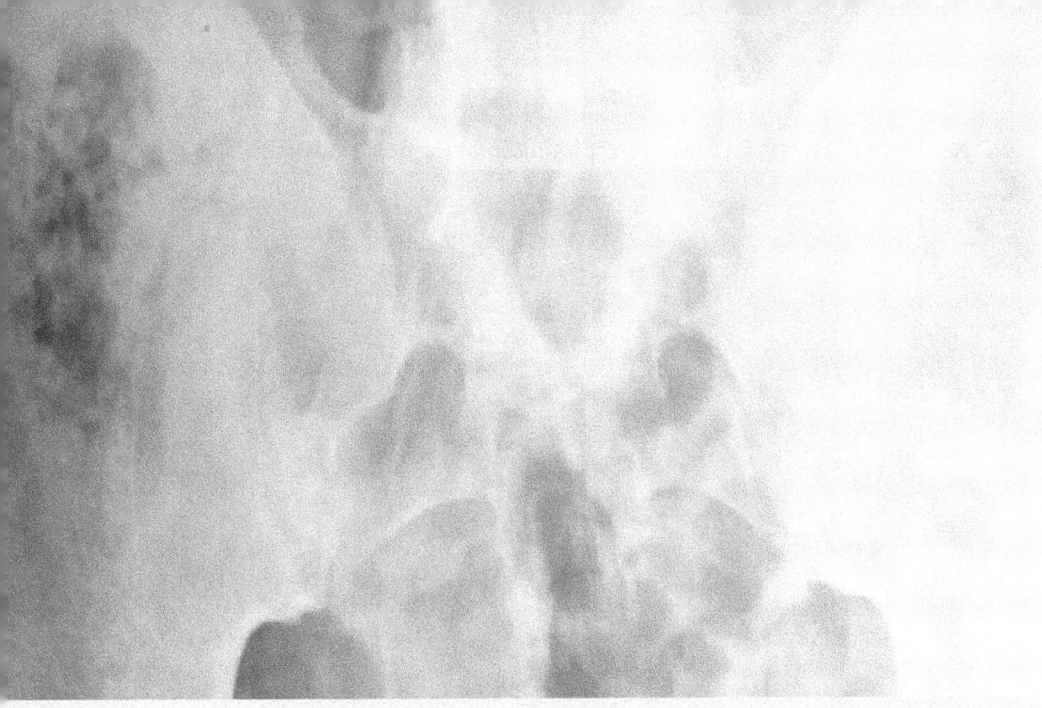

HIP JOINT ARTHRITIS AND AVASCULAR NECROSIS OF HIP

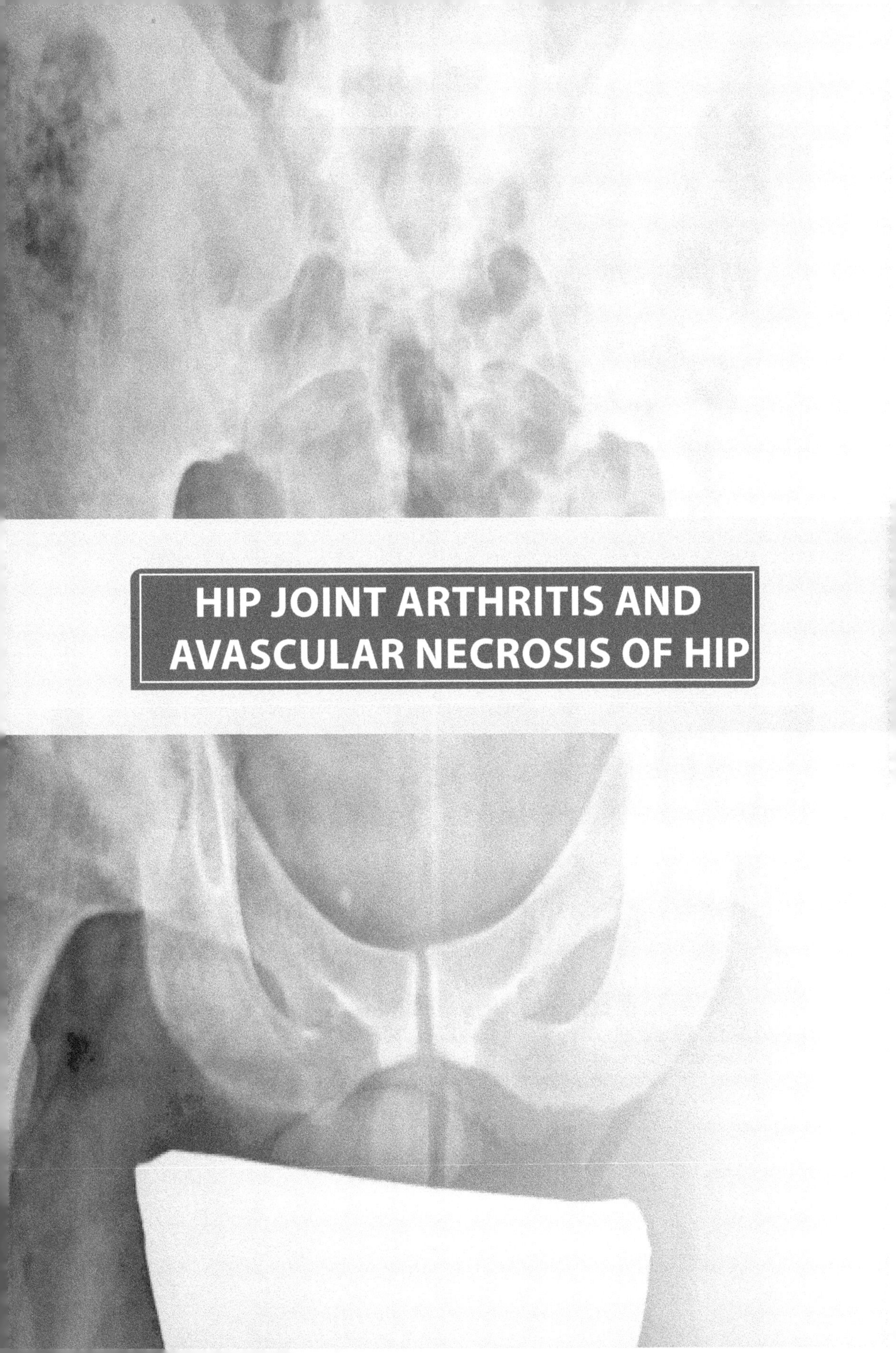

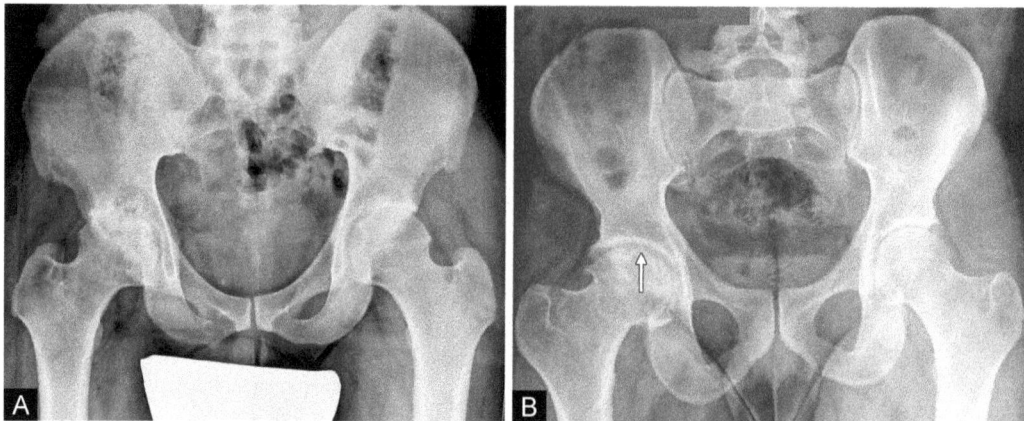

Figs. 73A and B: (A) Radiograph of pelvis, anteroposterior projection of a young male with advanced ankylosing spondylitis, showing reduced joint space in both hip joints with cortical irregularity in right hip joint. The findings are suggestive of hip joint damage due to arthritis. Note is also made of bilateral grade-3 sacroiliitis; (B) Radiograph of pelvis, anteroposterior projection of a young male with history of prolonged glucocorticoid use for scleritis showing crescent shaped radiolucency in the subarticular portion of head of right femur suggestive of avascular necrosis (white arrow). Unlike A, hip joint space width and sacroiliac joints are normal.

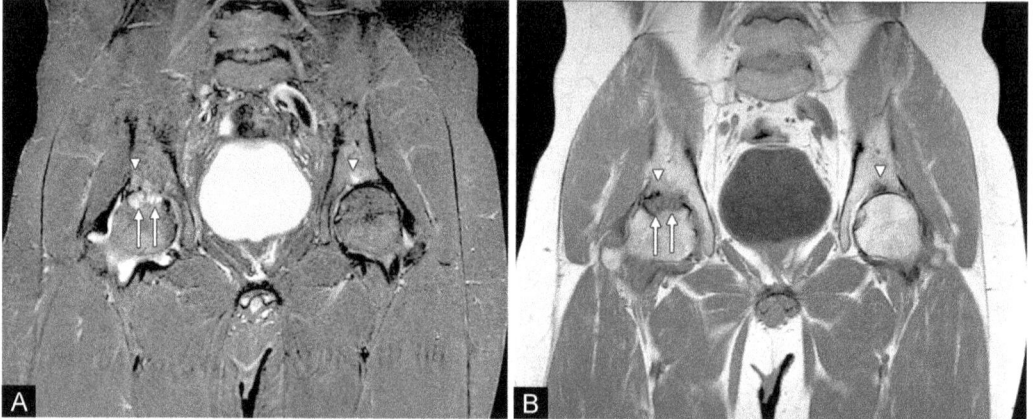

Figs. 74A and B: MRI of SIJ, coronal sections of a young male with advanced ankylosing spondylitis, showing bright signal intensity in the subarticular area of head of right femur (white arrows) and acetabulum on both sides (white arrowheads) on STIR sequence (A). Corresponding areas show dark signal intensities on T1W sequence (B). These features are typical of erosions which suggest hip joint arthritis.

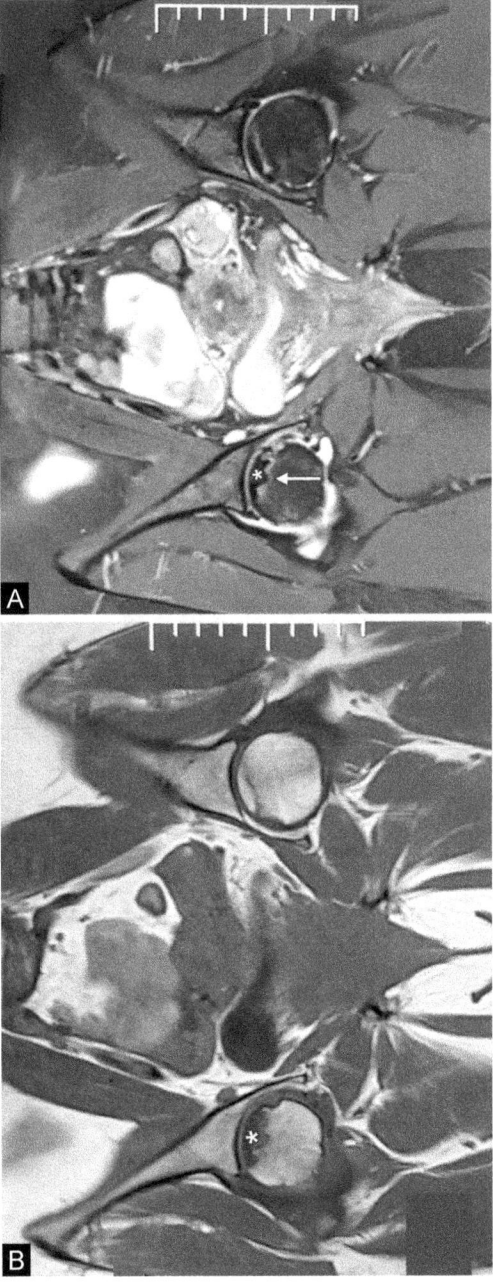

Figs. 75A and B: MRI of SIJ, coronal sections of a patient with granulomatosis with polyangiitis on long-term glucocorticoids, showing dark signal intensity in the subarticular area of head of right femur (asterisk) on both STIR (A) and T1W (B) sequences. Hip joint space is maintained and acetabulum is spared. Note the rim of bright signal intensity in the periphery of the dark area on STIR (arrow in A), with a typical 'serpiginous' contour. The features are suggestive of avascular necrosis (AVN) of hip. Compare the changes from those in hip arthritis (Figure 74). Joint space is compromised early in hip arthritis, as opposed to AVN. Erosions of the bone appear bright on STIR and dark on T1W sequences unlike AVN, which appears dark on both sequences.

CT SCAN

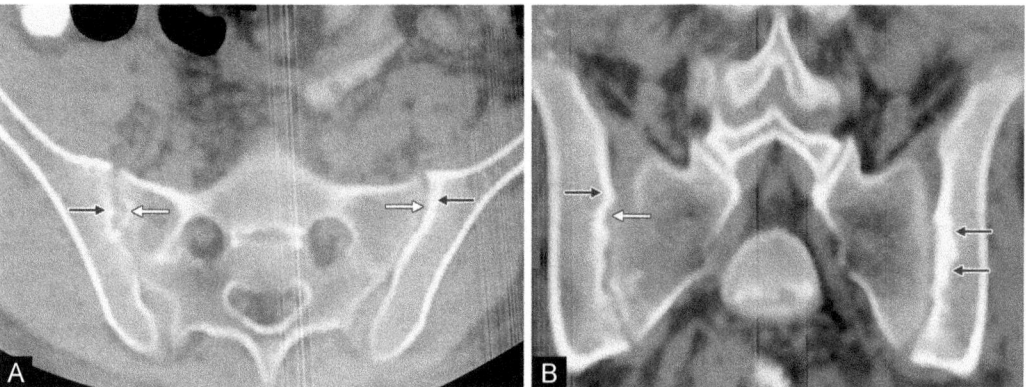

Figs. 76A and B: Computed tomography (CT) of pelvis showing sclerosis (black arrows) and erosions (white arrows) in both SIJ (A: axial section; B: coronal section).

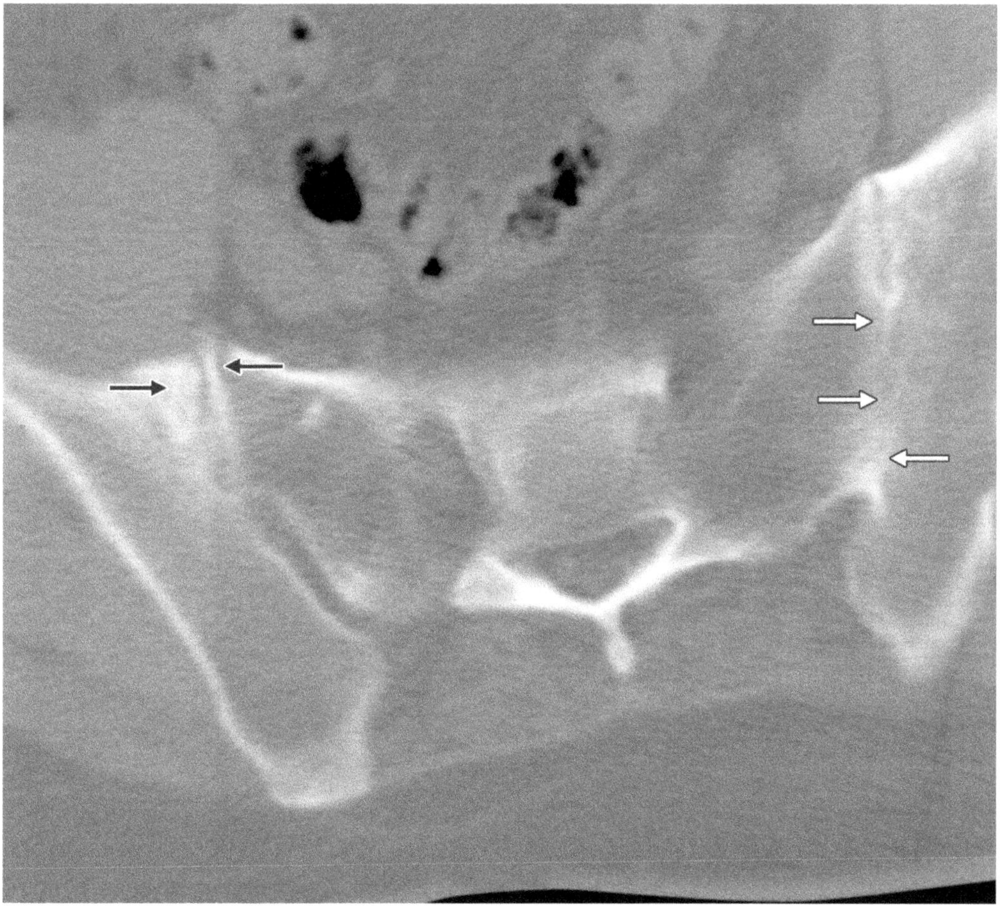

Fig. 77: Axial section of CT scan of SIJ showing obliteration of the joint space of left SIJ (ankylosis) (white arrows) and sclerosis of joint margins in right SIJ (black arrows).

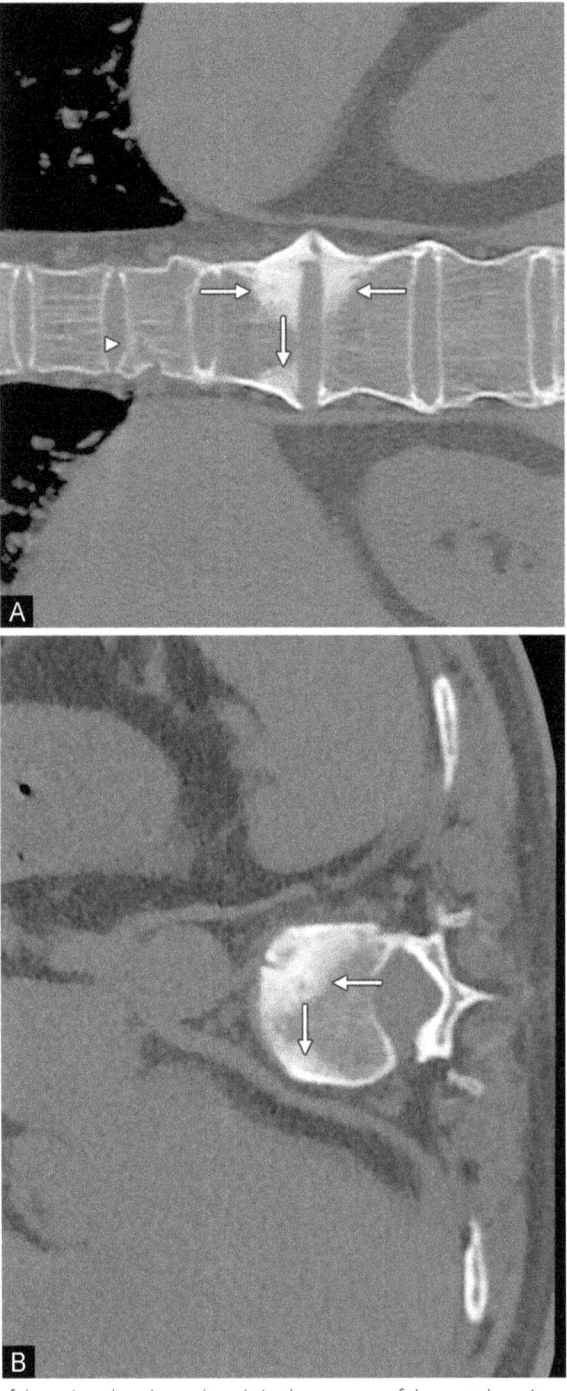

Figs. 78A and B: CT scan of the spine showing sclerosis in the corners of the vertebrae in coronal section in (A) (white arrows). Corresponding areas of sclerosis of vertebral body in axial section in (B) (white arrows). Multiple bridging and non-bridging syndesmophytes are seen in (A). Indentation of superior end-plate of T11 is also seen, suggestive of morphometric fracture (white arrowhead).

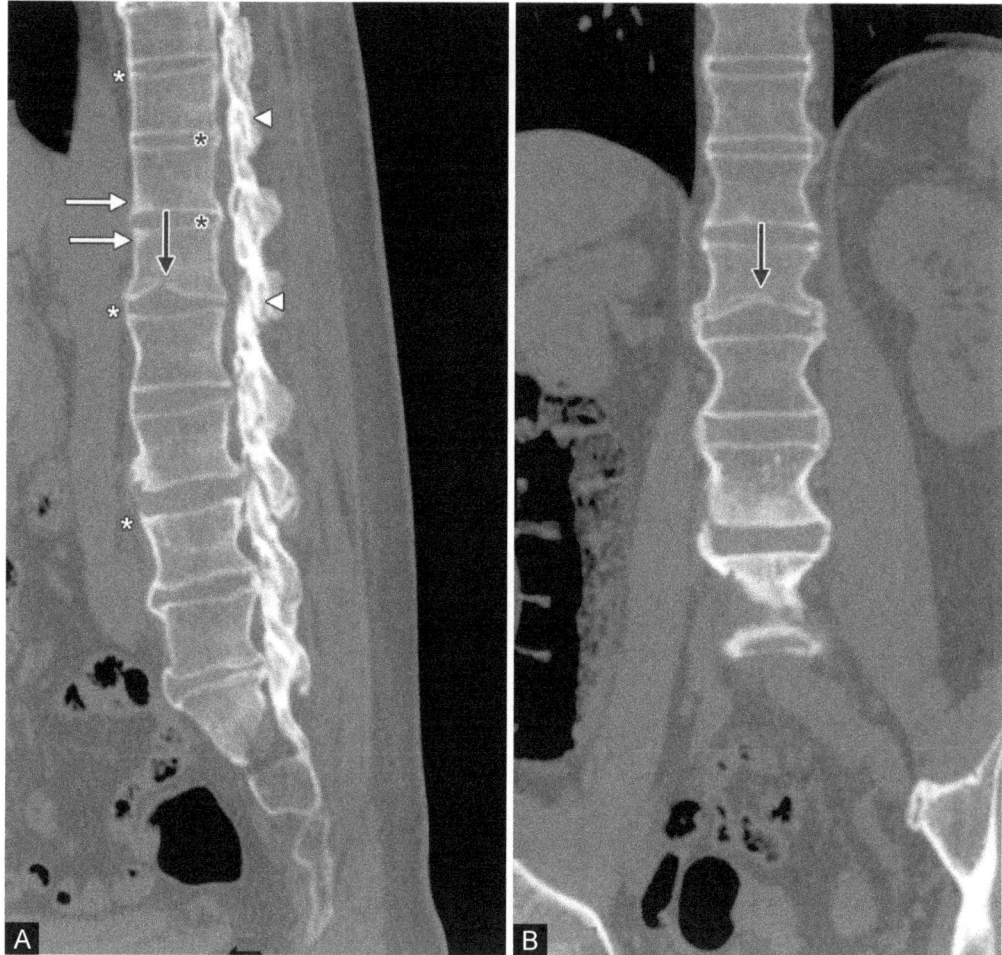

Figs. 79A and B: Computed tomography of the spine. (A) Sagittal section of thoracolumbar spine showing bridging and non-bridging syndesmophytes at multiple levels, both anteriorly (white asterisks) and posteriorly (black asterisks); sclerosis of lower anterior corner of T12 and upper anterior corner of L1, suggestive of 'shiny' corners (white arrows); break in the inferior end-plate of L1, suggestive of a morphometric fracture (black arrow) and sclerosis of facet joints (white arrowheads); (B) Coronal section of the same patient showing multiple syndesmophytes and fracture of the inferior end-plate of L1 vertebral body (black arrow).

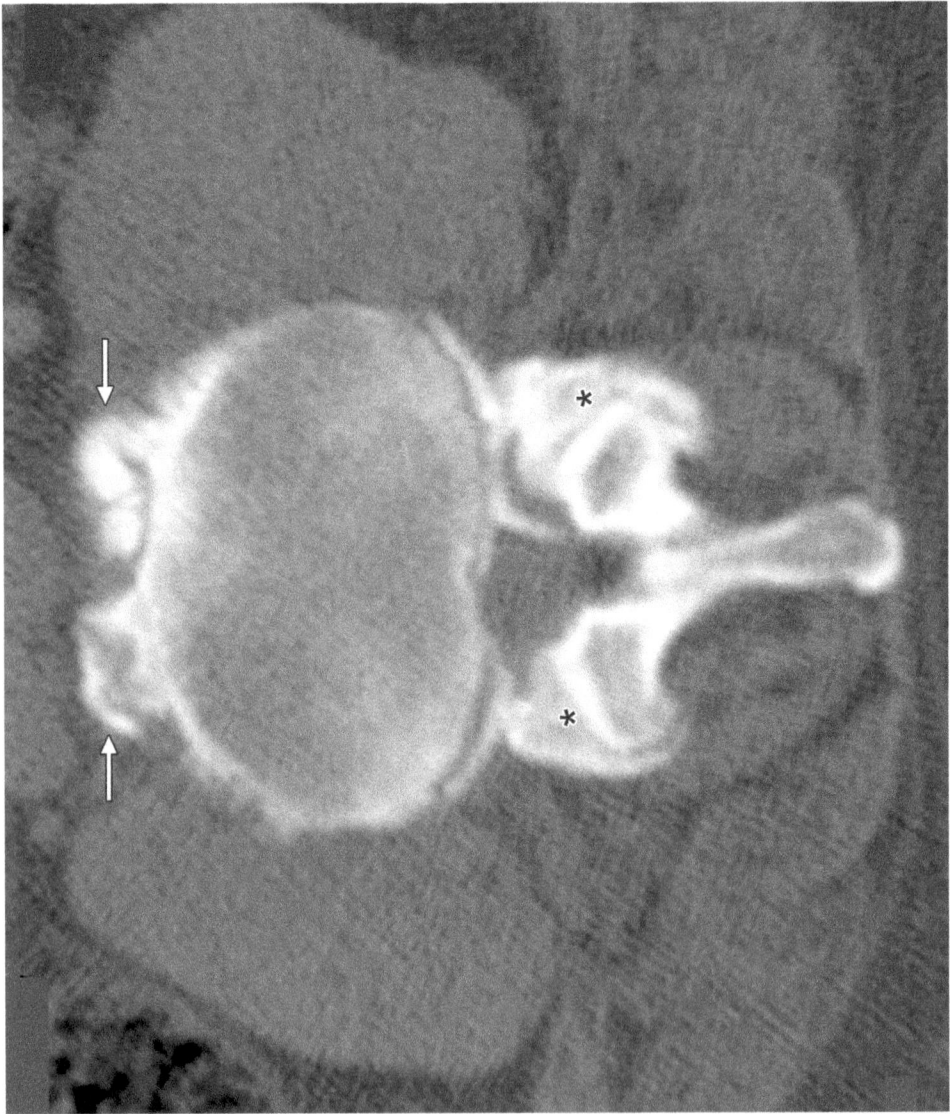

Fig. 80: CT scan, axial section of a patient with advanced, long-standing AS showing calcification anterior to the vertebral body, which corresponds to the area of anterior longitudinal ligament (ossification of anterior longitudinal ligament) (white arrows) and sclerosis of both facet joints (black asterisks).

ABBREVIATIONS

AFB: Acid fast bacillus
AS: Ankylosing spondylitis
ASAS: Assessment of Spondyloarthritis International Society
AVN: Avascular necrosis
CSF: Cerebrospinal fluid
CT: Computed tomography
ESSG: European Spondyloarthropathy Study Group criteria
IBP: Inflammatory back pain
JIA: Juvenile idiopathic arthritis
MRI: Magnetic resonance imaging
mSASSS: Modified Stoke Ankylosing Spondylitis Spine Score
OALL: Ossification of anterior longitudinal ligament
PCR: Polymerase chain reaction
SIJ: Sacroiliac joint
SpA: Spondyloarthritis
STIR: Short tau inversion recovery
T1W: T1 weighted
T2W: T2 weighted
ZN: Ziehl-Neelsen

REFERENCES

1. van der Linden S, Valkenburg HA, Cats A. Evaluation of diagnostic criteria for ankylosing spondylitis. A proposal for modification of the New York criteria. Arthritis Rheum. 1984;27:361-8.
2. Amor B, Dougados M, Mijiyawa M. Criteres de classification des spondylarthropathies. Rev Rhum Mal Osteoartic. 1990;57:85-9.
3. Dougados M, van der Linden S, Juhlin R, Huitfeldt B, Amor B, Calin A, et al. The European Spondylarthropathy Study Group preliminary criteria for the classification of spondylarthropathy. Arthritis Rheum. 1991;34:1218-27.
4. Rudwaleit M, van der Heijde D, Landewe´ R, Listing J, Akkoc N, Brandt J, et al. The development of Assessment of SpondyloArthritis international Society classification criteria for axial spondyloarthritis (part II): validation and final selection. Ann Rheum Dis. 2009;68:777-83.
5. Sieper J, van der Heijde D. Review: nonradiographic axial spondyloarthritis. new definition of an old disease? Arthritis Rheum. 2013;65:543-51.
6. Maksymowych WP, Lambert RG, Østergaard M, Pedersen SJ, Machado PM, Weber U, et al. MRI lesions in the sacroiliac joints of patients with spondyloarthritis: update of definitions and validation by the ASAS MRI working group. Ann Rheum Dis. 2019;78:1550-8.
7. Herregods N, Dehoorne J, Jaremko J, Joos R, Baraliakos X, Verstraete K, et al. Diagnostic value of MRI of the sacroiliac joints in juvenile spondyloarthritis. J Belg Soc Radiol. 2016;100:95.
8. Battistone MJ, Manaster BJ, Reda DJ, Clegg DO. Radiographic diagnosis of sacroiliitis—are sacroiliac views really better? J Rheumatol. 1998;25:2395-401.
9. Creemers MC, Franssen MJ, van't Hof MA, Gribnau FW, van de Putte LB, van Riel PL. Assessment of outcome in ankylosing spondylitis: an extended radiographic scoring system. Ann Rheum Dis. 2005;64:127-9.
10. Sieper J, Rudwaleit M, Baraliakos X, Brandt J, Braun J, Burgos-Vargas R, et al. The Assessment of SpondyloArthritis international Society (ASAS) handbook: a guide to assess spondyloarthritis. Ann Rheum Dis. 2009;68(Suppl II):ii1-ii44.
11. Maksymowych WP. The role of MRI in the evaluation of spondyloarthritis: a clinician's guide. Clin Rheumatol. 2016;35:1447-55.
12. Dale K. Radiographic grading of sacroiliitis in Bechterew's syndrome and allied disorders. Scand J Rheumatol. 1980;(supple 32):92.
13. Hermann KG, Althoff CE, Schneider U, Zühlsdorf S, Lembcke A, Hamm B, et al. Spinal changes in patients with spondyloarthritis: comparison of MR imaging and radiographic appearances. Radiographics. 2005;25:559-69.
14. Romanus R, Ydén S. Destructive and ossifying spondylitic changes in rheumatoid ankylosing spondylitis (Pelvo-spondylitis Ossificans). Acta Orthop Scand. 1952;22(2):88-99.
15. Mandl P, Navarro-Compán V, Terslev L, Aegerter P, van der Heijde D, D'Agostino MA, et al. EULAR recommendations for the use of imaging in the diagnosis and management of spondyloarthritis in clinical practice. Ann Rheum Dis. 2015;74:1327-39.
16. Aydingoz U, Yildiz AE, Ozdemir ZM, Yildirim SA, Erkus F, Ergen FB. A critical overview of the imaging arm of the ASAS criteria for diagnosing axial spondyloarthritis: what the radiologist should know. Diagn Interv Radiol. 2012;18:555-65.

EU GSPR Authorised Reprsentative
Logos Europe, 9 rue Nicolas Poussin
1700, La Rochelle, France
Phone: +33 (0) 6 67 93 73 78
E-mail: contact@logoseurope.eu

www.ingramcontent.com/pod-product-compliance
Ingram Content Group UK Ltd.
Pitfield, Milton Keynes, MK11 3LW, UK
UKHW060932280126
467427UK00008B/99